The **Cortisol Fix** Recipe Book

Reduce stress and bring your body back into balance with over 100 nourishing recipes

Angela Dowden

hamlyn

hamlyn

First published in Great Britain in 2024 by Hamlyn,
an imprint of
Octopus Publishing Group Ltd
Carmelite House
50 Victoria Embankment
London EC4Y 0DZ
www.octopusbooks.co.uk

An Hachette UK Company
www.hachette.co.uk

This material was previously published in *HAC: 10 Minute
Meals*, *HAC: 200 Easy Tagines & More*, *HAC: 200 Easy
Vegetarian*, *HAC: 200 Gluten-free Recipes*, *HAC: 200
Healthy Feasts*, *HAC: 200 Light Gluten-free*, *HAC: 200
One Pot Meals*, *HAC: 200 Super Salads*, *HAC: Tagines
& Moroccan Dishes*, *HAC: 200 Tapas & Spanish Dishes*,
HAC: 200 Vegan Recipes and *HAC: 200 Veggie Feasts*.

Distributed in the US by
Hachette Book Group
1290 Avenue of the Americas
4th and 5th Floors
New York, NY 10104

Distributed in Canada by
Canadian Manda Group
664 Annette St.
Toronto, Ontario, Canada M6S 2C8

ISBN 978-0-600-63884-1

A CIP catalogue record for this book is available from
the British Library.

Printed and bound in China.

10 9 8 7 6 5 4 3 2 1

Commissioning Editor: Louisa Johnson
Creative Director: Jonathan Christie
Editor: Scarlet Furness
Deputy Picture Manager: Jennifer Veall
Production Manager: Caroline Alberti

Standard level spoon measurements are used in all
recipes.
1 tablespoon = one 15 ml spoon
1 teaspoon = one 5 ml spoon

Both imperial and metric measurements have been given
in all recipes. Use one set of measurements only and not a
mixture of both.

Eggs should be medium unless otherwise stated. The
Department of Health advises that eggs should not be
consumed raw. This book contains dishes made with raw
or lightly cooked eggs. It is prudent for more vulnerable
people such as pregnant and nursing mothers, the elderly,
babies and young children to avoid uncooked or lightly
cooked dishes made with eggs. Once prepared these
dishes should be kept refrigerated and used promptly.

Milk should be full fat unless otherwise stated.

Fresh herbs should be used unless otherwise stated.
If unavailable use dried herbs as an alternative but halve
the quantities stated.

Ovens should be preheated to the specific temperature
– if using a fan-assisted oven, follow manufacturer's
instructions for adjusting the time and the temperature.

Pepper should be freshly ground black pepper unless
otherwise stated.

This book includes dishes made with nuts and nut
derivatives. It is advisable for those with known allergic
reactions to nuts and nut derivatives and those who
may be potentially vulnerable to these allergies, such as
pregnant and nursing mothers, the elderly, babies and
children, to avoid dishes made with nuts and nut oils.
It is also prudent to check the labels of pre-prepared
ingredients for the possible inclusion of nut derivatives.

Vegetarians should look for the 'V' symbol on a cheese
to ensure it is made with vegetarian rennet.

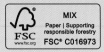

Contents

Introduction

Cortisol is an essential hormone with many important roles in the body. But if we consistently produce too much of it – usually as a response to chronic stress – our health will begin to suffer.

Feeling wired but tired and struggling to manage your weight are typical signs of cortisol overload. It's probably symptoms such as these that made you pick up this book in the first place. Doing so was a good move, as diet is key for keeping high cortisol and associated symptoms under control.

The Cortisol Fix Recipe Book will walk you through the foods and dietary patterns that can help to reduce excess cortisol. It will also touch on the complementary lifestyle actions that help ease chronic stress. The recipes that follow are rich in nutrients that support healthy stress hormone production, and the four-week planner is designed to ease you into your cortisol-curbing journey.

The following recipes are delicious and simple to create. So, in just a few short weeks, you can start moving the needle on high cortisol levels, without adding more stress to your life.

What is cortisol?

Cortisol is a hormone produced by the two adrenal glands, one located on top of each kidney. Part of a class of steroid hormones known as glucocorticoids, cortisol plays a crucial role in regulating our stress response, metabolism and immune system activity.[1]

In healthy people, cortisol is released according to a circadian rhythm, tying into our sleep-wake cycle. Levels are generally highest when we wake up and then fall throughout the day (if we work nights, this pattern is reversed). In between times, our cortisol levels will have mini surges depending on the stresses we deal with on any given day.

THE HPA AXIS

Cortisol levels move up and down via a feedback loop known as the hypothalamic-pituitary-adrenal (HPA) axis. This starts with the hypothalamus in the brain releasing a hormone called corticotropin-releasing hormone (CRH), which signals the pituitary gland to produce adrenocorticotropic hormone (ACTH). ACTH circulates to the adrenal glands, which in turn release cortisol. When cortisol levels peak, the hypothalamus stops releasing CRH and the feedback loop is complete.

It's a complex and sensitive setup designed to help us stay sharp and focused but may cause health issues if overwhelmed.

CORTISOL FUNCTIONS

When the HPA axis is working as it should, cortisol is our friend, with key functions that include:

- **Helping regulate blood glucose.** The hormone increases blood sugar levels, ensuring the body and brain have a ready supply of energy, especially during times of stress or fasting.
- **Damping down inflammation.** Cortisol can suppress some aspects of immune function, which helps control inflammation, and prevents the immune system from overreacting.
- **Regulating blood pressure.** Cortisol influences blood pressure by affecting the action of blood vessels and the heart. It can increase blood pressure to ensure adequate blood flow during stress.
- **Boosting brain function.** Cortisol affects memory, mood and behaviour. It plays a role in the sleep-wake cycle (rising when we wake and dipping later in the day). It also boosts cognitive responses to stress.

Cortisol and the fight-or-flight response

Another way to think of cortisol is as the body's built-in alarm system, alerting us to situations that require increased alertness and energy.

Cortisol is one of the main hormones in the fight-or-flight response, with adrenaline (epinephrine) being another.

When we face a physical or psychological stressor, this triggers a hormonal cascade that results in the adrenals secreting cortisol.

Cortisol then prepares the body for fight or flight by flooding it with glucose, which is an immediate energy source for muscles. Cortisol also narrows the arteries while epinephrine increases heart rate, which forces blood to pump harder and faster.

In ancient times you might have needed to deal with acute, short-term stressors like fleeing from a bear. These days though, many stressors tend to be chronic but longer term, such as long working hours or money worries. Sometimes chronically raised cortisol levels can also be due to traumatic events and abuse.[2]

This means we can't quickly resolve the cause of stress, and our bodies rarely revert to a fully relaxed state. Instead, we stay in a state of heightened alert, pumping out cortisol almost constantly.

FLATLINING CORTISOL

Sometimes the result of too much stress or trauma can take the form of a flattened cortisol curve rather than a chronically raised level. This means that the normal circadian rhythm of cortisol release is blunted or disrupted; for example, there isn't such a large morning peak, and levels don't fall off as much during the day.

In some cases, cortisol levels can stay permanently lower than normal with very little up or down movement at all. This so-called flatlining of cortisol has been seen in Holocaust survivors and victims of sexual abuse and may be an extreme response to a highly stressful environment.

Researchers believe that in these survivors, cortisol receptors may be extra sensitive to compensate. They also think that the same dietary and lifestyle steps that work for people with chronically raised cortisol work ultimately for flatliners too.

The health effects of disrupted cortisol

Chronically high or otherwise abnormal cortisol levels are implicated in all the following health issues. (Note: Cushing's disease is a separate medical condition involving very high cortisol levels and is not within our scope here).

CORTISOL AND DIABETES RISK

One of the ways cortisol readies us for fight or flight is by blocking the action of insulin – the hormone that pulls glucose out of our bloodstream into the muscles and liver. This raises the possibility that being over-exposed to cortisol can create insulin resistance, which often leads to type 2 diabetes.[3]

In people who already have type 2 diabetes, there is a clear link between increased cortisol levels and higher blood sugar levels.[4]

CORTISOL AND CARDIOVASCULAR CONDITIONS

Higher evening and early morning levels of cortisol have been associated with an increased risk of developing or dying from cardiovascular disease, as well as an increased risk of stroke.[5,6]

This might be because of the way cortisol and other stress hormones constrict our blood vessels, increasing our heart rate and blood pressure. Though this is helpful for fight-or-flight situations, over time these actions can lead to blood vessel damage and plaque buildup.

CORTISOL AND WEIGHT GAIN

High cortisol levels lead to increased appetite, which increases the chance of weight gain.

Researchers found that people who overproduced cortisol as a stress response in an experimental setting were more likely to snack when facing microaggressions in their regular lives.[7]

Cortisol may also be behind why we crave fatty, sugary foods when stressed. In one study, eating sugar reduced the amount that cortisol rose following stress exposure, suggesting we are driven to comfort eating to try to alleviate the detrimental effects of stress.[8]

More worryingly cortisol-related weight gain tends to be around the stomach,[9] which poses a greater heart disease and diabetes risk.

CORTISOL, IMMUNE ABNORMALITIES AND INFLAMMATION

Cortisol plays an important role in our immune systems, keeping inflammation under control so our immune responses aren't too reactive.

However, chronically high cortisol levels can lead to the immune system becoming resistant to cortisol's effects. This can cause an *increase* in the production of inflammatory chemicals, which stops our immune systems from working correctly.[10]

People with high cortisol levels are likely to suffer from more regular or more persistent infections, including common colds.[11]

CORTISOL AND MENTAL HEALTH

An elevated cortisol response is associated with acute and severe – but not mild – forms of clinical depression.[12]

In one scientific meta-analysis, adolescents with unusually high nocturnal cortisol levels were more likely to develop clinical depression in the future.[13]

However, it should be noted that it's likely to be caused by a more complex relationship than just cortisol causing depression.

One scientific review found that in women it was having a *variable* cortisol response to stress, rather than having high baseline cortisol, that correlated with depression.

CORTISOL AND SLEEP DISORDERS

Excessive activation of the cortisol-producing HPA axis appears to disrupt sleep, and likewise, sleep disruptions can also increase cortisol levels. This suggests that abnormalities within the cortisol production control centre may play a role in both starting and prolonging chronic insomnia.

That said, the cortisol-sleep relationship is complex and not fully understood. It may be that high cortisol levels in the evening and when falling asleep are a marker for certain brain activities with the potential to disrupt sleep, rather than the direct cause of insomnia.[14]

How diet can help balance cortisol levels

There is no one perfect cortisol-lowering diet. But, a diet that feeds the healthy bacteria in your microbiome, helps to fight inflammation and is balanced (with a plant focus) is likely to be very helpful.

Let's look at how these three healthy eating principles can benefit your cortisol levels, before moving on to specific nutrients that may help.

NOURISH YOUR MICROBIOME

Research suggests a link between stress and the bacteria that make up your gut microbiome. Fostering a healthy and diverse gut microbiome could help lower cortisol levels and reduce the impact of stress.

Kombucha, sauerkraut, kimchi, live yogurt, kefir and other fermented drinks are all probiotic foods (rich in friendly gut bacteria) that can boost your gut microbiome, so ideally include some of these in your diet when trying to reduce your cortisol level.

In one study, cortisol levels reduced significantly in students who drank a daily probiotic drink for 12 weeks, compared to a control group. Another study suggested a link between probiotic foods and reduced social anxiety.[15]

Similarly, *prebiotics* are essential for good gut health, which may then go on to positively impact stress and cortisol levels.

Instead of containing bacteria, prebiotics are plant fibres that feed friendly bacteria already in the gut. Garlic, onions, leeks, asparagus, Jerusalem artichokes, oats, bananas and seeds (like flax and chia) are all good sources of prebiotics that can boost levels of good bacteria such as Bifidobacteria.

EAT TO QUELL INFLAMMATION

High levels of background inflammation in the body can lead to cortisol overload as the hormone remains switched on in an attempt to damp down the excess inflammation.

Eating an anti-inflammatory diet means cortisol levels will tend to decline as there is less work for the hormone to do. An anti-inflammatory diet will usually have these hallmarks:

- Low glycemic load (less fast-releasing sugar and refined carbs, more whole food carbs like whole grains, pulses and so on)
- Low in saturated fats and trans fatty acids (such as fatty processed meats and takeaways)
- Rich in vitamins, minerals and phytochemicals (from foods like nuts, berries and vegetables)
- High in fibre
- Low in alcohol

In one study involving over 200 teenagers, researchers found that those who ate a Mediterranean diet (which is an example of an anti-inflammatory diet), had lower cortisol levels than the participants who didn't.[16]

EAT BALANCED (MAINLY PLANTS)

Becoming vegan or vegetarian isn't necessary but leaning towards more plant-based proteins like beans, lentils and tofu makes sense when watching your cortisol levels.

One study measured cortisol levels in the adult offspring of 1970s mothers who had been advised to eat lots of red meat and avoid carbohydrates during pregnancy. It noted a 5 per cent increase in cortisol concentration for each portion of maternal animal protein eaten daily – in short, a large intake of red meat resulted in higher cortisol levels in the next generation.

Cutting carbs is also not helpful for managing high cortisol. Research in overweight and obese women showed that eating more wholegrain carbohydrates as part of a healthy diet helped lower cortisol levels.[17] Low-fat dairy may also help keep cortisol in check,[18] while fasting increases levels.[19]

The takeaway point is that balanced eating (in line with current dietary guidelines) is better than any kind of fad when managing your cortisol levels.

3 top cortisol-lowering nutrients

While it's our diet as a whole that counts most, some specific nutrients are worth seeking out when we're looking to balance our cortisol levels.

OMEGA-3S

Anti-inflammatory omega-3 fats found naturally in oily fish can help reduce raised cortisol levels. One study linked high cortisol levels in the evening with low blood levels of omega-3s.[20]

In another study, when nurses received omega-3 supplements, cortisol levels decreased, and feelings of burnout, including emotional exhaustion, also lessened.[21] We can get a meaningful amount of omega-3s from consuming about two portions of oily fish (salmon, trout, sardines, mackerel) weekly.

FLAVANOLS

Many fruits, vegetables and pulses provide flavanols, which are phytochemicals that may help to optimize cortisol function in the face of stress.[22] However green tea and cocoa beans are the best sources.

We only need to drink two-and-a-half cups of green tea daily to provide the full 500 milligrams of flavanols deemed beneficial, whereas we'd need to eat four apples or six cups of blueberries to get the same amount.

Natural, non-alkalized cocoa powder is also a great source of flavanols (check for acidity regulators, such as potassium carbonate, in the ingredients, as this is a sign that the cocoa has been alkalized so won't be such a potent flavanol source). Dark chocolate contains some flavanols but can't be relied on as a good source, as flavanols can be destroyed during bean-to-bar processing.

MAGNESIUM

Several studies suggest that the mineral magnesium – which many of us don't get enough of – plays a role in preventing high cortisol levels.[23]

Magnesium may also help people feel less anxious, but properly designed and controlled trials are still lacking on this topic.[24] The best magnesium sources are almonds, Brazils and other nuts, along with pulses, green leafy vegetables, wholemeal bread and other wholegrains.

Caffeine and cortisol levels

Tea, coffee and chocolate are all sources of caffeine which has been shown to increase cortisol levels.[25]

However, caffeine also enhances brain processing speeds and seems to protect against depression,[26] so there are pros and cons to consider before giving up a coffee habit.

The deciding factor will usually be how many cups of caffeinated drink you have currently and whether you feel dependent on your daily brew.

A practical guide could be to stick to no more than two cups a day and have these in the morning to coincide with when you would expect your cortisol level to be higher anyway. If you currently consume a lot of caffeine, cut down slowly.

Cutting caffeine out altogether isn't generally necessary though. Coffee and tea (both green and black) can protect against cardiovascular conditions and some cancers,[27, 28] so can be good for your longer-term health.

Curbing your cortisol with lifestyle changes

Changing your diet and using the recipes and eating plans in this book can be really helpful in controlling cortisol levels. But dietary measures work best when they go hand-in-hand with lifestyle changes that reduce stress.

Which practices you find most successful in managing stress will depend on your preferences and time demands. But here are a few lifestyle tweaks to try.

PRACTICE MEDITATION-MINDFULNESS

Incorporating these relaxation practices into your daily routine can help you develop greater resilience to stress. Effective meditation-mindfulness practice can be as simple as focusing on your in-out breathing for a few minutes as you sit somewhere quiet and comfortable. Apps like Headspace can be helpful to guide you.

ENLIST HERBAL HELP

One small study found that taking ashwagandha, a traditional Indian herb available in health foods shops, significantly reduced levels of cortisol and improved sleep.[29]

Another small study had similar findings, with ashwagandha reportedly decreasing stress levels, improving memory and focus, and boosting psychological well-being.[30]

BE PHYSICALLY ACTIVE

The best exercise to beat stress is the one you like doing best, as this will help you stick to it.

Vigorous exercise results in a short-term spike of cortisol but improves your cortisol response to later stressful events. Try not to do intense cardio exercise like running or a spin class late in the evening though – this might be a better time for something more calming like restorative yoga.

ENGAGE IN YOUR FAVOURITE HOBBIES

Spending time on activities that bring you joy can offer a welcome break from stress and worry.

HEAD OUT INTO NATURE

Even short exposure to green spaces can help. In one study, scientists showed that when people spent just twenty minutes in 'urban nature' – leafy streets or a park for example – levels of salivary cortisol dropped. It didn't matter what sort of activity they were doing at the time.[31]

IMPROVE YOUR SLEEP HYGIENE

Eating healthily, exercising and engaging in relaxation practices are fundamental to improving sleep. Other sleep hygiene practices that will help curb your cortisol levels include having a set bedtime and waking time, and making sure your bedroom is quiet, dark and a comfortable temperature, with no phones or tablets by the bed.

BIBLIOGRAPHY

1   Thau L, Gandhi J, Sharma S. Physiology, Cortisol. StatPearls. Treasure Island (FL): StatPearls Publishing; 2024.

2   Elzinga BM, Schmahl CG, Vermetten E, van Dyck R, Bremner JD. Higher cortisol levels following exposure to traumatic reminders in abuse-related PTSD. Neuropsychopharmacology. 2003 Sep;28(9):1656–65.

3   Joseph JJ, Golden SH. Cortisol dysregulation: the bidirectional link between stress, depression, and type 2 diabetes mellitus. Ann N Y Acad Sci. 2017 Mar;1391(1):20–34.

4   Dias JP, Joseph JJ, Kluwe B, Zhao S, Shardell M, Seeman T, et al. The longitudinal association of changes in diurnal cortisol features with fasting glucose: MESA. Psychoneuroendocrinology. 2020 Sep;119:104698.

5   Karl S, Johar H, Ladwig K-H, Peters A, Lederbogen F. Dysregulated diurnal cortisol patterns are associated with cardiovascular mortality: Findings from the KORA-F3 study. Psychoneuroendocrinology. 2022 Jul;141:105753.

6   Crawford AA, Soderberg S, Kirschbaum C, Murphy L, Eliasson M, Ebrahim S, et al. Morning plasma cortisol as a cardiovascular risk factor: findings from prospective cohort and Mendelian randomization studies. Eur J Endocrinol. 2019 Oct;181(4):429–38.

7   Newman E, O'Connor DB, Conner M. Daily hassles and eating behaviour: the role of cortisol reactivity status. Psychoneuroendocrinology. 2007 Feb;32(2):125–32.

8   Di Polito N, Stylianakis AA, Richardson R, Baker KD. Real-world intake of dietary sugars is associated with reduced cortisol reactivity following an acute physiological stressor. Nutrients. 2023 Jan 1;15(1).

9   Moyer AE, Rodin J, Grilo CM, Cummings N, Larson LM, Rebuffé-Scrive M. Stress-induced cortisol response and fat distribution in women. Obes Res. 1994 May;2(3):255–62.

10 Vitlic A, Lord JM, Phillips AC. Stress, ageing and their influence on functional, cellular and molecular aspects of the immune system. Age (Dordr). 2014 Jun;36(3):9631.

11 Cohen S, Janicki-Deverts D, Doyle WJ, Miller GE, Frank E, Rabin BS, et al. Chronic stress, glucocorticoid receptor resistance, inflammation, and disease risk. Proc Natl Acad Sci USA. 2012 Apr 17;109(16):5995–9.

12 Nandam LS, Brazel M, Zhou M, Jhaveri DJ. Cortisol and major depressive disorder-translating findings from humans to animal models and back. Front Psychiatry. 2019;10:974.

13 Zajkowska Z, Gullett N, Walsh A, Zonca V, Pedersen GA, Souza L, et al. Cortisol and development of depression in adolescence and young adulthood – a systematic review and meta-analysis. Psychoneuroendocrinology. 2022 Feb;136:105625.

14 Hirotsu C, Tufik S, Andersen ML. Interactions between sleep, stress, and metabolism: From physiological to pathological conditions. Sleep Sci. 2015 Nov;8(3):143–52.

15 Hilimire MR, DeVylder JE, Forestell CA. Fermented foods, neuroticism, and social anxiety: An interaction model. Psychiatry Res. 2015 Aug 15;228(2):203–8.

16 Carvalho KMB, Ronca DB, Michels N, Huybrechts I, Cuenca-Garcia M, Marcos A, et al. Does the Mediterranean diet protect against stress-induced inflammatory activation in European adolescents? The HELENA Study. Nutrients. 2018 Nov 15;10(11).

17 Soltani H, Keim NL, Laugero KD. Increasing dietary carbohydrate as part of a healthy whole food diet intervention dampens eight week changes in salivary cortisol and cortisol responsiveness. Nutrients. 2019 Oct 24;11(11).

18 Witbracht MG, Van Loan M, Adams SH, Keim NL, Laugero KD. Dairy food consumption and meal-induced cortisol response interacted to influence weight loss in overweight women undergoing a 12-week, meal-controlled, weight loss intervention. J Nutr. 2013 Jan;143(1):46–52.

19 Nakamura Y, Walker BR, Ikuta T. Systematic review and meta-analysis reveals acutely elevated plasma cortisol following fasting but not less severe calorie restriction. Stress. 2016 Jan 7;19(2):151–7.

20 Thesing CS, Bot M, Milaneschi Y, Giltay EJ, Penninx BWJH. Omega-3 polyunsaturated fatty acid levels and dysregulations in biological stress systems. Psychoneuroendocrinology. 2018 Nov;97:206–15.

21 Jahangard L, Hedayati M, Abbasalipourkabir R, Haghighi M, Ahmadpanah M, Faryadras M, et al. Omega-3-polyunsatured fatty acids (O3PUFAs), compared to placebo, reduced symptoms of occupational burnout and lowered morning cortisol secretion. Psychoneuroendocrinology. 2019 Nov;109:104384.

22 Ruijters EJB, Haenen GRMM, Weseler AR, Bast A. The cocoa flavanol (-)-epicatechin protects the cortisol response. Pharmacol Res. 2014 Jan; 79:28–33.

23 Cuciureanu MD, Vink R. Magnesium and stress. In: Vink R, Nechifor M, editors. Magnesium in the Central Nervous System. Adelaide (AU): University of Adelaide Press; 2011.

24 Boyle NB, Lawton C, Dye L. The Effects of Magnesium Supplementation on Subjective Anxiety and Stress-A Systematic Review. Nutrients. 2017 Apr 26;9(5).

25 Lovallo WR, Farag NH, Vincent AS, Thomas TL, Wilson MF. Cortisol responses to mental stress, exercise, and meals following caffeine intake in men and women. Pharmacol Biochem Behav. 2006 Mar;83(3):441–7.

26 Grosso G, Micek A, Castellano S, Pajak A, Galvano F. Coffee, tea, caffeine and risk of depression: A systematic review and dose-response meta-analysis of observational studies. Mol Nutr Food Res. 2016 Jan;60(1):223–34.

27 Poole R, Kennedy OJ, Roderick P, Fallowfield JA, Hayes PC, Parkes J. Coffee consumption and health: umbrella review of meta-analyses of multiple health outcomes. BMJ. 2017 Nov 22;359:j5024.

28 Khan N, Mukhtar H. Tea and health: studies in humans. Curr Pharm Des. 2013;19(34):6141–7.

29 Salve J, Pate S, Debnath K, Langade D. Adaptogenic and anxiolytic effects of ashwagandha root extract in healthy adults: A double-blind, randomized, placebo-controlled clinical study. Cureus. 2019 Dec 25;11(12):e6466.

30 Gopukumar K, Thanawala S, Somepalli V, Rao TSS, Thamatam VB, Chauhan S. Efficacy and safety of ashwagandha root extract on cognitive functions in healthy, stressed adults: A randomized, double-blind, placebo-controlled study. Evid Based Complement Alternat Med. 2021 Nov 30;2021:8254344.

31 Hunter MR, Gillespie BW, Chen SY-P. Urban nature experiences reduce stress in the context of daily life based on salivary biomarkers. Front Psychol. 2019 Apr 4;10:722.

Meal Plans

Here you will find four weekly meal plans to get you started with your healthy cortisol-lowering diet. Your main meals should include at least two or three portions of vegetables or salad, so add extra where necessary. A portion is about what you can hold in your palm, and any non-starchy, steamed, boiled or stir-fried vegetable counts, as does a bowlful of mixed leaves. The Green Salad on page 56 or Roasted Summer Vegetables on page 58 work great as extra sides.

In terms of drinks, try to consume herbal teas (green tea is especially beneficial), coffee (though not if you are caffeine-sensitive) and plenty of water.

Week 1

	Breakfast	Lunch	Dinner	Snacks
Monday	Porridge with semi-skimmed milk, topped with berries, chopped almonds & a drizzle of honey	Orange & Avocado Salad (see page 76)	Chickpea & Aubergine Tagine (see page 134)	Handful of Moroccan-style Spiced Chickpeas (see page 90); one apple
Tuesday	Egg-filled Mushrooms on Toast (see page 40)	Beans & Peppers with Harissa (see page 184) with a slice of wholegrain bread	Baked salmon served with stir-fried vegetables, wholewheat noodles & a splash of soy sauce	Handful of unsalted nuts; mini easy peeler such as a clementine or satsuma
Wednesday	Goats' Cheese Omelettes (see page 22); glass of orange juice	Butter Bean & Tomato Soup (see page 162) with toasted sourdough	Grilled chicken served with Veg Kebabs (see page 112) and spinach; Cheese & Paprika Potato Cakes (see page 170)	Greek-style Feta & Mint Dip (see page 108) with carrot & cucumber sticks
Thursday	Lemon, Pistachio & Fruit Squares (see page 46); handful of blueberries	Baked sweet potato stuffed with sautéed spinach & crumbled feta	Mackerel Curry (see page 142) with brown rice	Handful of Citrus Olives (see page 88) with feta cubes
Friday	Smashed avocado on sourdough, topped with a poached egg	Canned sardines on toasted sourdough; handful of cherry tomatoes	Chicken & Barley Risotto (see page 140)	Handful of Moroccan-style Spiced Chickpeas (see page 90); one apple
Saturday	Honey Roasted Granola (see page 28) with Greek yogurt & a handful of mixed berries	Raspberry Salad with Toasties (see page 82)	Vegetable Broth & Sea Bass (see page 136) with boiled new potatoes	One apple; a few squares of dark chocolate
Sunday	Lemon, Pistachio & Fruit Squares (see page 46); glass of orange juice	Smoked Trout & Grape Salad (see page 78)	Chicken & Pickled Walnut Pilaf (see page 138)	Handful of unsalted nuts; one nectarine

Week 2

	Breakfast	Lunch	Dinner	Snacks
Monday	Mixed Mushrooms on Toast (see page 24)	Wholegrain wrap with cold shredded roast chicken, avocado, lettuce & hummus	Turkey Chilli (see page 122)	Couple of Wholemeal Cheese Straws (see page 114); handful of cherry tomatoes
Tuesday	Quinoa Porridge with Raspberries (see page 35)	Grilled Salmon with Kale Salad (see page 152)	Stir-fry made with colourful veg, one chicken breast, wholewheat noodles & a splash of soy sauce	One apple; a few squares of dark chocolate
Wednesday	Sourdough toast topped with reduced-fat cream cheese & smoked salmon; bowl of berries	Baked sweet potato topped with avocado, salsa & lime juice	Moroccan-style Fish Tagine (see page 150); Green Beans with Almonds (see page 179)	Pepper & Aubergine Hummus (see page 100) served on two rye crispbreads
Thursday	Honey Roasted Granola (see page 28) with Greek yogurt & a handful of mixed berries	Bang Bang Chicken Salad (see page 53)	Two grilled chicken thighs with Moroccan-style Vegetable Couscous (see page 156)	Handful of unsalted nuts; one nectarine
Friday	Porridge with semi-skimmed milk, topped with nut butter, blueberries & a drizzle of honey	Chicken & Hummus Wraps (see page 163); handful of cherry tomatoes	Artichoke & Asparagus Pizzas (see page 148)	Handful of Citrus Olives (see page 88) with feta cubes
Saturday	Spinach, Feta & Egg Tarts (see page 26); glass of orange juice	Pepper & Aubergine Hummus (see page 100) served on two rye crispbreads; one banana	Harissa Salmon with Sweet Potato (see page 126)	One apple; a few squares of dark chocolate
Sunday	Pancakes with Blueberry Sauce (see page 30)	Moroccan-style Vegetable Couscous (see page 156)	Chicken with Spinach & Ricotta (see page 128) with new potatoes	Pepper & Aubergine Hummus (see page 100) served on two rye crispbreads

Week 3

	Breakfast	Lunch	Dinner	Snacks
Monday	Shredded wheat served with semi-skimmed milk, chopped banana & chopped nuts	Ginger Chicken Soup (see page 168) served with a slice of wholegrain bread	Grilled salmon with quinoa served with Spicy Roasted Cherry Tomatoes (see page 182)	Greek-style Feta & Mint Dip (see page 108) with carrot & cucumber sticks
Tuesday	Soft-boiled Eggs with Harissa (see page 25); handful of mixed berries	Leftover, chilled Spicy Roasted Cherry Tomatoes (see page 182) with mozzarella and a slice of wholegrain bread	Mediterranean Roasted Fish (see page 132) served with wholewheat couscous	One apple; a few squares of dark chocolate
Wednesday	Smashed avocado on sourdough, topped with a poached egg	Smoked Trout & Grape Salad (see page 78)	Chickpea & Aubergine Tagine (see page 134)	Handful of unsalted nuts; mini easy peeler such as a clementine or satsuma
Thursday	Smoothie made with ½ banana, big handful of strawberries, 1 tablespoon of nut butter & 150 ml (¼ pint) plant-based or dairy milk	Hot Haloumi with Fattoush Salad (see page 54)	Penne with Peas & Beans (see page 124)	Smoked Trout & Horseradish Pâté (see page 102) with crackers
Friday	Mixed Mushrooms on Toast (see page 24)	Canned sardines on toasted sourdough with sliced cucumber & carrot	Turkish-style Stuffed Butternut Squash (see page 146)	Apple slices with nut butter
Saturday	Quinoa Porridge with Raspberries (see page 35)	Aubergine with Caper & Mint Dressing (see page 180)	Speedy Spiced Chicken Tagine (see page 144)	Natural or Greek yogurt with a handful of mixed berries
Sunday	Potato Farls with Mushrooms (see page 20)	Salmon & Cucumber Sushi (see page 172)	Steak with skin-on potato wedges, served with rocket & Parmesan flakes tossed in balsamic vinegar & olive oil	Handful of Citrus Olives (see page 88) with feta cubes

Week 4

	Breakfast	Lunch	Dinner	Snacks
Monday	Breakfast Cereal Bars (see page 34); handful of blueberries	Baked sweet potato stuffed with sautéed spinach & crumbled feta	Two grilled chicken thighs with Moroccan-style Vegetable Couscous (see page 156)	Smoked Trout & Horseradish Pâté (see page 102) with crackers
Tuesday	Smoothie made with ½ banana, big handful of strawberries, 1 tablespoon of nut butter & 150 ml (¼ pint) plant-based or dairy milk	Buckwheat & Salmon Salad (see page 52)	Roasted Stuffed Peppers (see page 176) served with quinoa	Natural or Greek yogurt with a handful of mixed berries
Wednesday	Breakfast Cereal Bars (see page 34); glass of orange juice	Wholegrain wrap with cold shredded roast chicken, avocado, lettuce & hummus	Turkey Chilli (see page 122)	Couple of Wholemeal Cheese Straws (see page 114); handful of cherry tomatoes
Thursday	Goats' Cheese Omelettes (see page 22)	Bang Bang Chicken Salad (see page 53)	Pasta with Fennel & Rocket (see page 131)	One apple; a few squares of dark chocolate
Friday	Shredded wheat, served with semi-skimmed milk, chopped banana & chopped nuts	Chicken & Hummus Wraps (see page 163); carrot sticks	Baked salmon served with stir-fried vegetables, wholewheat noodles & a splash of soy sauce	Handful of Citrus Olives (see page 88) with mini mozzarella balls
Saturday	Pancakes with Blueberry Sauce (see page 30)	Butter Bean & Tomato Soup (see page 162) with toasted sourdough	Chicken & Pickled Walnut Pilaf (see page 138)	Handful of unsalted nuts; mini easy peeler such as a clementine or satsuma
Sunday	Spinach, Feta & Egg Tarts (see page 26); handful of blueberries	Salmon & Sesame Skewers (see page 115); bowl of salad leaves	Mango & Coconut Curry (see page 130)	Greek-style Feta & Mint Dip (see page 108) with carrot & cucumber sticks

Breakfast

- **SERVES: 4**
- **PREPARATION TIME: 10 MINUTES**
- **COOKING TIME: 25 MINUTES**

TIP

Canning increases the availability of the lycopene in tomatoes – a healthy phytochemical that can reduce cell damage and has been linked with better heart health.

Spicy Tomato Poached Eggs

2 tablespoons olive oil

1 onion, finely chopped

2 garlic cloves, crushed

1 teaspoon sweet smoked paprika

1 thyme sprig

2 x 400 g (13 oz) cans chopped tomatoes

200 ml (7 fl oz) water

4 eggs

salt and pepper

chopped parsley, to garnish

Heat the oil in a large, deep frying pan, add the onion and cook for 5 minutes until softened. Stir in the garlic and paprika and cook for a further 30 seconds.

Add the thyme sprig, tomatoes and the measurement water, then season with salt and pepper. Bring to the boil, then reduce the heat and simmer for 10 minutes until rich and thickened.

Make 4 small pockets in the tomato sauce, then break an egg into each one. Cover the pan with foil and simmer for about 5 minutes until the egg whites are cooked through. Serve scattered with chopped parsley.

- **FOR HEARTY TOMATO VEGETABLE STEW WITH EGGS**

Heat 3 tablespoons olive oil in a frying pan, add 1 chopped aubergine and fry until golden. Remove from the pan and set aside. Add 1 cored, deseeded and chopped red pepper and more oil, if needed, to the pan and fry until softened. Remove from the pan and set aside. Make the sauce as above, adding the reserved aubergines and pepper to the pan with the tomatoes. Continue as above.

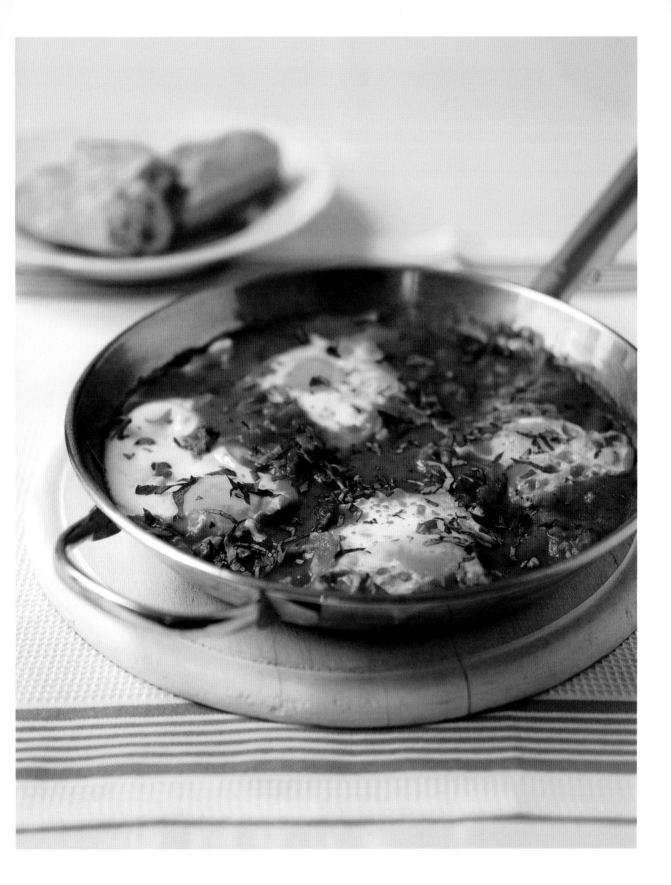

- **SERVES: 2**
- **PREPARATION TIME: 15 MINUTES**
- **COOKING TIME: 12 MINUTES**

Potato Farls with Mushrooms

1 tablespoon olive oil

25 g (1 oz) unsalted butter

2 shallots, finely chopped

250 g (8 oz) mixed mushrooms, such as chestnut, portobello and button, trimmed and sliced

2 garlic cloves, chopped

1 tablespoon lemon juice

2 tablespoons chopped flat leaf parsley

2 large eggs

4 ready-made potato farls, toasted

salt and pepper

1 tablespoon chopped chives, to garnish

Heat the oil with the butter in a frying pan over a high heat. Reduce the heat slightly, add the shallots and mushrooms and fry for 6 minutes, stirring occasionally, until the mushrooms are golden. Stir in the garlic and cook, stirring, for 1 minute.

Add the lemon juice to the mushroom mixture and season with salt and pepper.

Remove the pan from the heat and stir in the parsley. Keep warm while you poach the eggs.

Half-fill a separate frying pan with water and bring to a simmer. Break in the eggs and cook for 3 minutes.

Place 2 potato farls on each warmed serving plate and top with the mushroom mixture, then the eggs. Sprinkle with the chives and serve immediately.

- **FOR POTATO RÖSTI WITH BAKED EGGS & TOMATOES**

Place 8 ready-made small frozen potato rösti in a roasting tin with 12 cherry tomatoes and drizzle with 1 tablespoon olive oil. Cook in a preheated oven, 200°C (400°F), Gas Mark 6, for 10 minutes. Remove from the oven and turn the röstis over. Return to the oven and cook for a further 6 minutes until golden. Break 2 eggs into the roasting tin and return to the oven for 2–3 minutes or until the eggs are just set. Place 4 rösti on each warmed serving plate, divide the roasted tomatoes between the plates and add a baked egg to each.

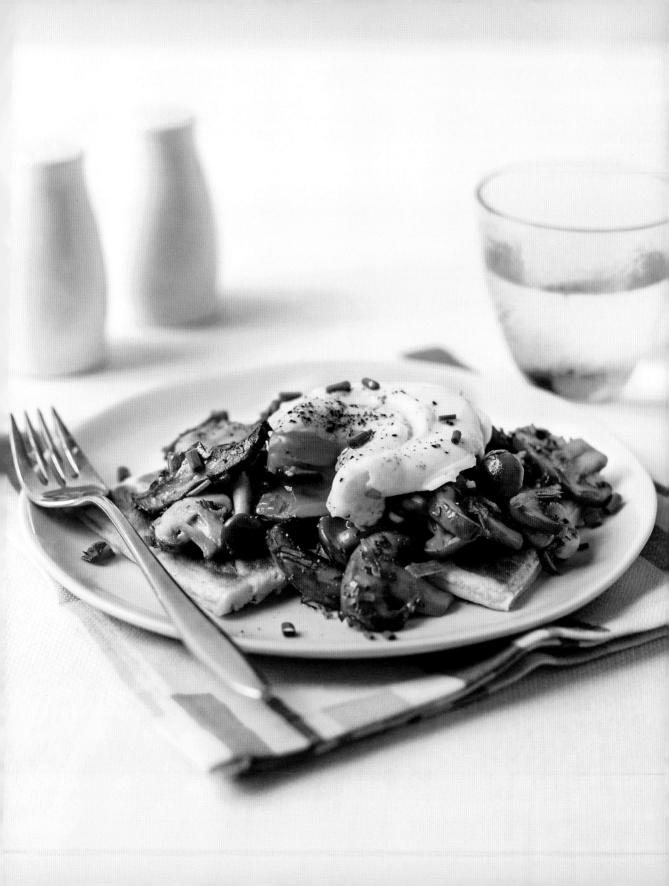

- **SERVES: 4**
- **PREPARATION TIME: 10 MINUTES**
- **COOKING TIME: 20 MINUTES**

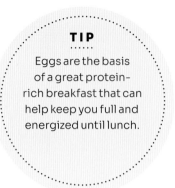

TIP

Eggs are the basis of a great protein-rich breakfast that can help keep you full and energized until lunch.

Goats' Cheese Omelettes

4 tablespoons olive oil

500 g (1 lb) mixed red and yellow cherry tomatoes, halved

a little basil, chopped, plus a few sprigs, to garnish

12 eggs

2 tablespoons wholegrain mustard

50 g (2 oz) butter

100 g (3½ oz) soft goats' cheese, diced

salt and pepper

watercress, to garnish

Heat the oil in a frying pan, add the tomatoes and cook over a medium heat for 2–3 minutes until softened (you may have to do this in 2 batches). Add the basil and season to taste with salt and pepper, then transfer to a bowl and keep warm.

Beat the eggs with the mustard in a large bowl and season with salt and pepper.

Melt one-quarter of the butter in an omelette pan or small frying pan over a medium heat until it stops foaming, then swirl in one-quarter of the egg mixture. Fork over the omelette so that it cooks evenly. As soon as it is set on the bottom (but still a little runny in the middle), dot over one-quarter of the goats' cheese and cook for a further 30 seconds. Carefully slide the omelette on to a warmed plate, folding it in half as you do so. Keep warm.

Repeat with the remaining mixture to make 3 more omelettes. Serve with the tomatoes, garnished with watercress and basil sprigs.

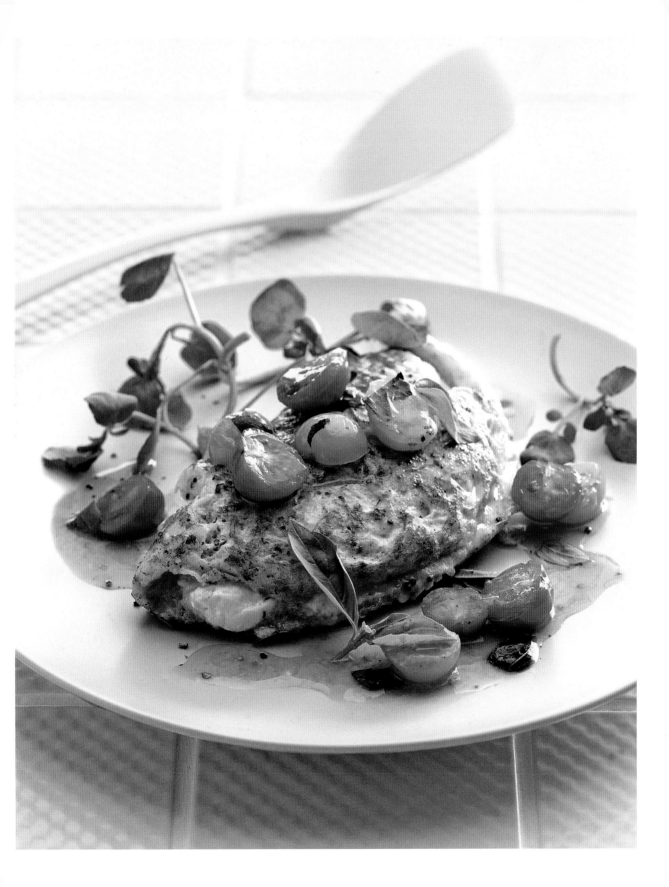

- **SERVES: 4**
- **PREPARATION TIME: 10 MINUTES**
- **COOKING TIME: 5 MINUTES**

TIP

Mushrooms provide the antioxidant, anti-inflammatory mineral selenium, along with B vitamins that help our bodies release energy from food.

Mixed Mushrooms on Toast

25 g (1 oz) butter

3 tablespoons extra virgin olive oil, plus extra to serve

750 g (1½ lb) mixed mushrooms, such as oyster, shiitake, flat and button, trimmed and sliced

2 garlic cloves, crushed

1 tablespoon chopped thyme

grated rind and juice of 1 lemon

2 tablespoons chopped parsley

4 slices of sourdough bread

100 g (3½ oz) mixed salad leaves

salt and pepper

fresh Parmesan cheese shavings, to serve

Melt the butter with the oil in a large frying pan. As soon as the butter stops foaming, add the mushrooms, garlic, thyme, lemon rind and salt and pepper and cook over a medium heat, stirring, for 4–5 minutes until tender. Scatter over the parsley, squeeze over a little lemon juice and stir in.

Meanwhile, toast the bread, then arrange it on serving plates.

Top the sourdough toast with the salad leaves and mushrooms, and drizzle over a little more oil and lemon juice. Scatter with Parmesan shavings and serve immediately.

- **FOR FIELD MUSHROOMS & CAMEMBERT ON TOAST**

Trim 8 large field mushrooms, brush with 2 tablespoons olive oil and cook under a preheated hot grill for 4–5 minutes on each side. Lightly toast 4 slices of sourdough bread, top with the mushrooms and arrange 2 slices of Camembert cheese over each one. Cook under the grill for 2–3 minutes until the cheese has melted then serve.

- **SERVES:** 4
- **PREPARATION TIME: 5 MINUTES**
- **COOKING TIME: 3–5 MINUTES**

Soft-boiled Eggs with Harissa

4 eggs

4 slices of wholemeal bread

4 heaped teaspoons ready-made harissa paste (for homemade harissa paste, see below)

Homemade chilli harissa paste

12 large fresh red chillies

3 tablespoons olive oil

1 teaspoon cumin seeds

1 teaspoon coriander seeds

1 teaspoon caraway or fennel seeds

3–4 garlic cloves, chopped

1 teaspoon salt

1 tablespoon finely chopped coriander

First, make the homemade harissa paste, if using. Place the chillies in an ovenproof dish, pour over the oil and roast in a preheated oven, 200°C (400°F), Gas Mark 6, for 20–25 minutes until the skins begin to buckle. Meanwhile, dry-fry all the seeds in a small, heavy-based frying pan over a medium heat for 2–3 minutes until they emit a nutty aroma, then grind in a spice grinder.

Using a small, sharp knife, remove the stalks and skins from the roasted chillies. Slit lengthways and scrape out the seeds. Using a pestle and mortar, pound the chilli flesh, garlic and salt to a smooth paste. Add the spices, mix with 2–3 tablespoons of the roasting oil and stir in the coriander. Spoon the harissa into a small bowl and drizzle over a little more roasting oil.

Next, prepare the eggs. Place the eggs in a saucepan of water, bring to the boil and cook for 3–5 minutes, depending on how you like your eggs. Meanwhile, toast the bread and cut into long strips.

Drain the eggs, cut them in half and serve on a plate with the strips of toast and a small bowl of harissa. To eat, first dip the strips of toast into the harissa, then dip into the egg.

- **MAKES: 4**
- **PREPARATION TIME: 15 MINUTES**
- **COOKING TIME: 16–18 MINUTES**

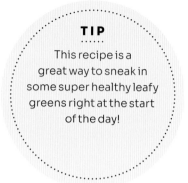

TIP

This recipe is a great way to sneak in some super healthy leafy greens right at the start of the day!

Spinach, Feta & Egg Tarts

250 g (8 oz) frozen leaf spinach, defrosted

125 g (4 oz) feta cheese, diced

2 tablespoons mascarpone cheese

pinch of freshly grated nutmeg

4 sheets of filo pastry, defrosted if frozen

50 g (2 oz) butter, melted

4 eggs

salt and pepper

Drain the spinach and squeeze out all the excess water, then chop finely. Place in a bowl and mix in the feta, mascarpone, nutmeg and salt and pepper to taste.

Lay the sheets of filo pastry on top of one another in a pile, brushing each with a little melted butter. Cut out 4 x 15 cm (6 inch) rounds using a saucer as a template.

Divide the spinach mixture between the pastry rounds, spreading the filling out but leaving a 2.5 cm (1 inch) border. Gather the edges of the pastry up and over the filling to form a rim. Make a shallow well in the spinach mixture.

Transfer the tarts to a baking sheet and bake in a preheated oven, 200°C (400°F), Gas Mark 6, for 8 minutes. Remove from the oven and carefully crack an egg into each hollow. Bake for a further 8–10 minutes until the eggs are set.

- **FOR SPINACH & GOATS' CHEESE PARCELS**

Prepare the spinach as above, then mix with 125 g (4 oz) soft goats' cheese, 2 tablespoons mascarpone cheese, a pinch of ground cumin and salt and pepper to taste. Cut out the filo pastry rounds as above and divide the spinach mixture between them, but place it on one half of each round. Carefully fold the pastry over the filling and turn the pastry edges over to seal. Bake in the oven as above and serve with lemon wedges for squeezing over and Greek yogurt.

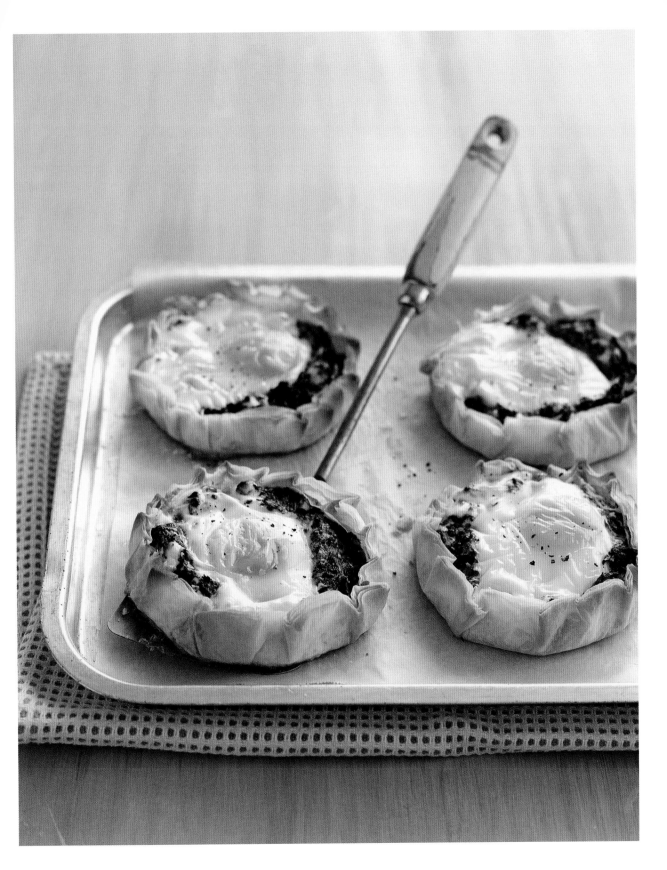

- **SERVES: 4**
- **PREPARATION TIME: 10 MINUTES, PLUS COOLING**
- **COOKING TIME: 25–30 MINUTES**

TIP

The nuts in this granola are a good source of magnesium for lowering cortisol and improving nerve and muscle health. They will also minimize the blood glucose spike you'll get from the sweeter ingredients.

Honey Roasted Granola

3 tablespoons clear honey

2 tablespoons sunflower oil

250 g (8 oz) porridge oats

50 g (2 oz) hazelnuts, roughly chopped

50 g (2 oz) blanched almonds, roughly chopped

50 g (2 oz) dried cranberries

50 g (2 oz) dried blueberries

To serve

skimmed milk or low-fat bio yogurt

fresh fruit

Heat the honey and oil together gently in a small saucepan.

Mix the oats and nuts together thoroughly in a large bowl. Pour over the warm honey mixture and stir well to combine.

Spread the mixture over a large nonstick baking sheet and bake in a preheated oven, 150°C (300°F), Gas Mark 2, for 20–25 minutes, stirring once, until golden.

Leave the granola to cool, then stir in the dried berries. Serve with skimmed milk or low-fat bio yogurt and fresh fruit. Any remaining granola can be stored in an airtight container.

- **FOR OVEN-BAKED CHOCOLATE, ALMOND & CHERRY GRANOLA**

Mix the warmed honey and sunflower oil as above with 2 tablespoons sifted cocoa powder. Mix the porridge oats and 100 g (3½ oz) blanched almonds together in a large bowl. Pour over the warm honey mixture and stir well to combine. Bake as above and leave to cool, then stir in 100 g (3½ oz) dried cherries. Serve with milk.

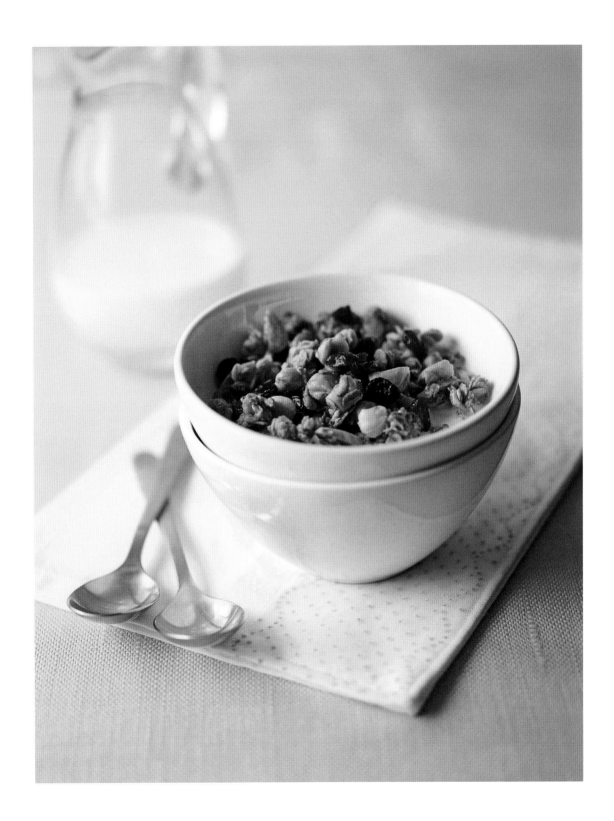

- SERVES: 4–6
- PREPARATION TIME: 10 MINUTES
- COOKING TIME: 20 MINUTES

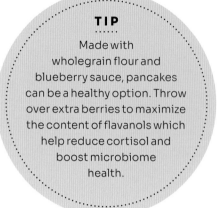

TIP

Made with wholegrain flour and blueberry sauce, pancakes can be a healthy option. Throw over extra berries to maximize the content of flavanols which help reduce cortisol and boost microbiome health.

Pancakes with Blueberry Sauce

15 g (½ oz) butter

150 g (5 oz) wholemeal self-raising flour

1 teaspoon bicarbonate of soda

40 g (1½ oz) caster sugar

1 egg, beaten

350 ml (12 fl oz) buttermilk

icing sugar, for dusting

Greek yogurt or crème fraîche, to serve

Blueberry sauce

250 g (8 oz) fresh blueberries

2 tablespoons clear honey

dash of lemon juice

For the blueberry sauce, heat the blueberries with the honey and lemon juice in a small saucepan over a low heat for about 3 minutes until they release their juices. Keep warm.

Melt the butter in a separate small saucepan. Sift the flour and bicarbonate of soda into a bowl and stir in the caster sugar. Beat the egg and buttermilk together in a separate bowl or jug, then gradually whisk into the dry ingredients with the melted butter to make a smooth batter.

Heat a nonstick frying pan until hot. Drop in large spoonfuls of the batter and cook over a high heat for 3 minutes until bubbles appear on the surface. Flip the pancakes and cook for a further minute. Remove and keep warm in a moderate oven. Repeat with the remaining batter.

Serve the pancakes topped with the blueberry sauce and Greek yogurt or crème fraîche and dusted with icing sugar.

- **FOR PANCAKES WITH SPICED APPLE SAUCE**

Replace the blueberries with 1 peeled, cored and chopped juicy dessert apple and use maple syrup instead of the honey, adding 1 teaspoon ground cinnamon, or to taste. Cook the pancakes as above and serve with the spiced apple sauce.

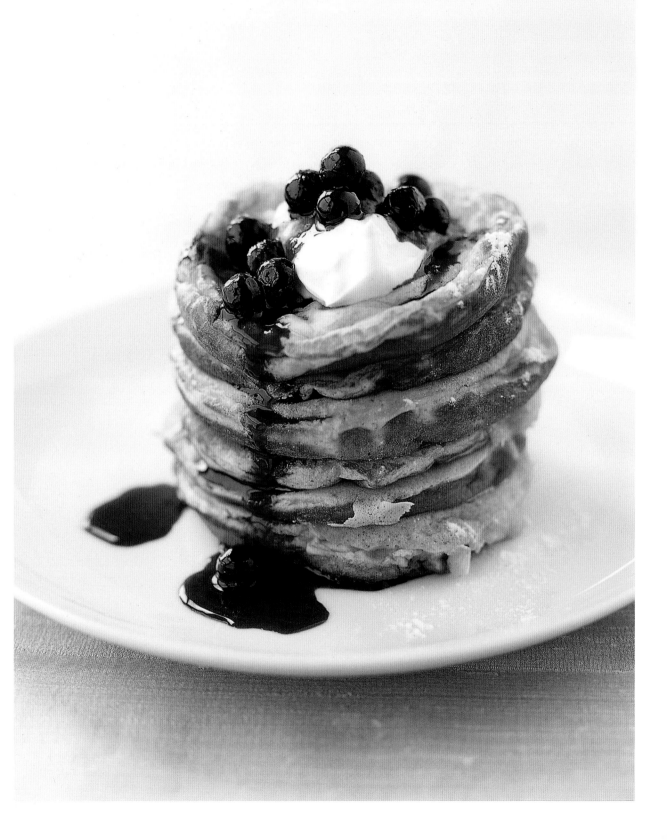

French Toast with Apple & Raspberry Sauce

2 eggs, beaten

1 teaspoon vanilla extract

100 ml (3½ fl oz) milk

1 tablespoon caster sugar

½ teaspoon ground cinnamon

4 thick slices of wholemeal bread or sourdough

25 g (1 oz) butter

Apple & raspberry sauce

25 g (1 oz) butter

6 eating apples, peeled, cored and sliced

1 tablespoon light soft brown sugar

½ teaspoon ground cinnamon

125 g (4 oz) raspberries

Whisk the eggs with the vanilla extract, milk, sugar and cinnamon in a shallow dish. Place the slices of bread in the mixture, turning to coat both sides so that they absorb the liquid.

Heat the butter in a nonstick frying pan. Use a palette knife or fish slice to transfer the soaked bread to the hot pan and fry for 2 minutes on each side until golden.

Meanwhile, for the apple and raspberry sauce, heat the butter in a frying pan, add the apples and fry for 2–3 minutes. Sprinkle over the soft light brown sugar, ground cinnamon and raspberries and cook gently for 1–2 minutes.

Cut the toasts in half diagonally, then pour over the sauce and serve immediately.

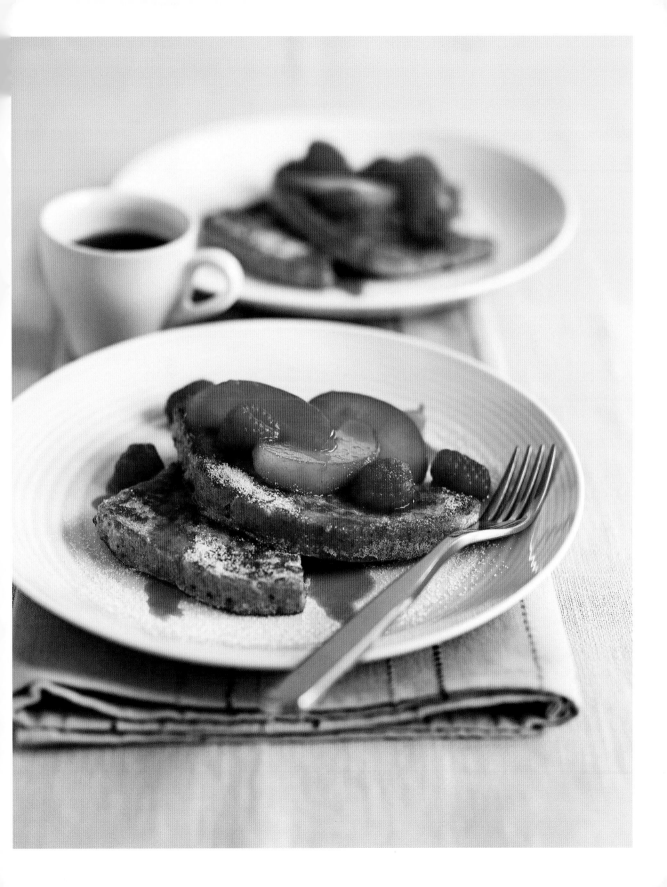

- **MAKES: 16**
- **PREPARATION TIME: 10 MINUTES**
- **COOKING TIME: 35 MINUTES**

TIP

Seeds are super rich in important minerals and elevate the nutritional value of this on-the-run breakfast option.

Breakfast Cereal Bars

100 g (3½ oz) butter, softened, plus extra for greasing

25 g (1 oz) soft light brown sugar

125 g (4 oz) millet flakes

50 g (2 oz) quinoa

50 g (2 oz) dried cherries or cranberries

75 g (3 oz) sultanas

25 g (1 oz) sunflower seeds

25 g (1 oz) sesame seeds

25 g (1 oz) linseeds

40 g (1½ oz) unsweetened desiccated coconut

2 eggs, lightly beaten

Grease a 28 x 20 cm (11 x 8 inch) shallow baking tin.

Beat together the butter and sugar in a large bowl until creamy. Add all the remaining ingredients and beat well until combined.

Spoon the mixture into the prepared tin, level the surface with the back of a dessertspoon and place in a preheated oven, 180°C (350°F), Gas Mark 4, for 35 minutes until deep golden. Remove from the oven and leave to cool in the tin.

Turn out on to a wooden board and carefully cut into 16 fingers using a serrated knife. Store in an airtight container for up to 5 days.

- **FOR YOGURTY CRUNCH**

Slice 2 bananas and divide half the slices between 4 tall glasses. Mix together 300 ml (½ pint) natural yogurt and 4 tablespoons runny honey in a bowl and spoon half the mixture over the slices. Crumble 4 Breakfast Cereal Bars (see above) and sprinkle half over the yogurt mixture. Repeat the layering, chill and serve.

- **SERVES: 2**
- **PREPARATION TIME: 5 MINUTES**
- **COOKING TIME: 25–30 MINUTES**

Quinoa Porridge with Raspberries

600 ml (1 pint) semi-skimmed milk

100 g (3½ oz) quinoa

2 tablespoons caster sugar

½ teaspoon ground cinnamon

125 g (4 oz) fresh raspberries

2 tablespoons mixed seeds, such as sunflower, linseed, pumpkin and hemp

Bring the milk to the boil in a small saucepan. Add the quinoa and return to the boil. Reduce the heat to low, cover and simmer for about 15 minutes until three-quarters of the milk has been absorbed.

Stir the sugar and cinnamon into the pan, re-cover and cook for 8–10 minutes or until almost all the milk has been absorbed and the quinoa is tender.

Spoon the porridge into 2 bowls, then top with the raspberries and sprinkle over the seeds. Serve immediately.

- **FOR QUINOA & MAPLE SYRUP PANCAKES**

Mix together 225 g (7½ oz) precooked quinoa, 1 large lightly beaten egg, 125 g (4 oz) plain fl our, 2 teaspoons baking powder, ½ teaspoon each of ground cinnamon and salt, 200 ml (7 fl oz) milk and 2 tablespoons maple syrup in a large bowl until well combined. Melt a little butter in a frying pan, add separate heaped tablespoonfuls of the batter and cook for 2–3 minutes on each side until golden brown. Serve with Greek yogurt and fresh berries.

- **SERVES: 4**
- **PREPARATION TIME: 5 MINUTES**
- **COOKING TIME: 5 MINUTES**

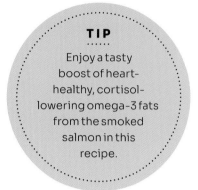

TIP

Enjoy a tasty boost of heart-healthy, cortisol-lowering omega-3 fats from the smoked salmon in this recipe.

Smoked Salmon Scrambled Eggs

8 eggs

2 tablespoons fromage frais

1 tablespoon chopped chives

125 g (4 oz) smoked salmon, cut into strips

salt and pepper

buttered toast, to serve (optional)

Whisk together the eggs, fromage frais and salt and pepper in a bowl.

Heat a saucepan over a medium heat, pour in the egg mixture and cook for 1 minute, then using a spatula, gently push the egg around to ensure it cooks evenly.

When the egg looks like creamy curds, stir in the chives and smoked salmon and serve immediately on buttered toast, if liked.

- **FOR SMOKED SALMON FRITTATA**

Thickly slice 500 g (1 lb) new potatoes and cook in a pan of boiling water for 8–10 minutes, then drain. Lightly beat 8 large eggs, then stir in 200 g (7 oz) strips of smoked salmon, 2 tablespoons chopped dill, 100 g (3½ oz) petits pois and the potatoes. Season. Heat 2 tablespoons olive oil in a frying pan with an ovenproof handle. Pour in the egg mixture and cook for 10–15 minutes over a low heat until the egg is starting to set. Place under a preheated medium grill and cook for 3–4 minutes, or until the egg is set and the top is golden. Turn out on to a board and cut into wedges to serve.

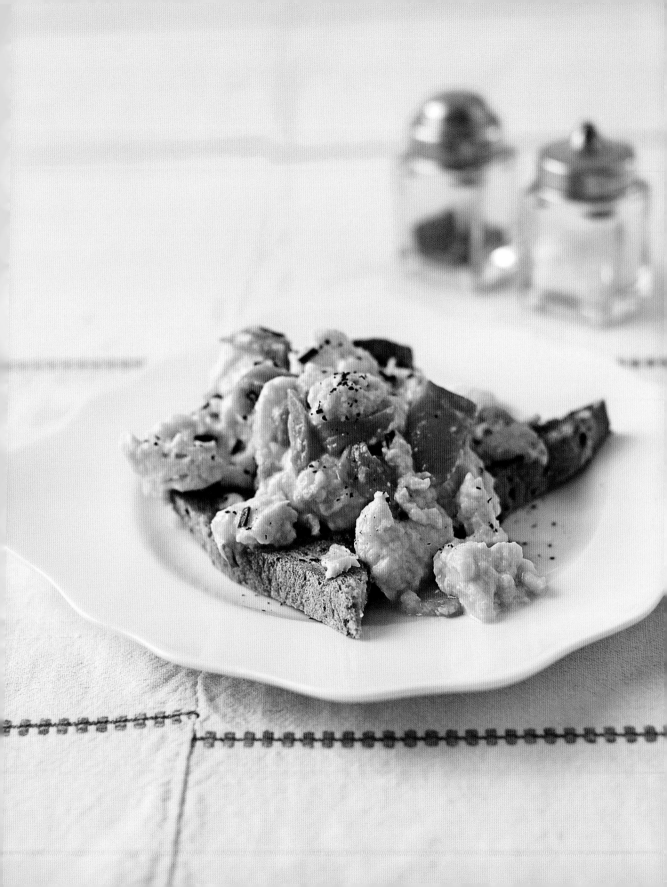

- MAKES: 12
- PREPARATION TIME: 10 MINUTES
- COOKING TIME: 10 MINUTES

Mini Tomato & Feta Omelettes

melted butter, for greasing

4 eggs, beaten

2 tablespoons chopped chives

3 sun-dried tomatoes, finely sliced

75 g (3 oz) feta cheese, crumbled

salt and pepper

Brush a 12-hole mini muffin tray lightly with melted butter to grease.

Mix together all the remaining ingredients in a large bowl until just combined.

Pour the mixture into the greased holes and place in a preheated oven, 220°C (425°F), Gas Mark 7, for about 10 minutes until golden and puffed up. Remove from the oven and serve warm.

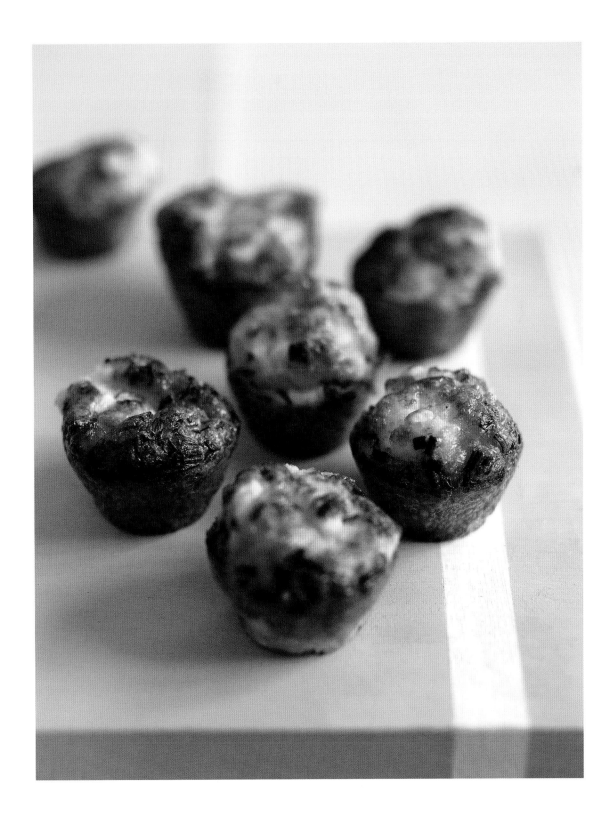

- **SERVES: 4**
- **PREPARATION TIME: 5 MINUTES**
- **COOKING TIME: 10-15 MINUTES**

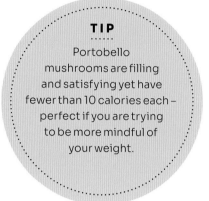

TIP

Portobello mushrooms are filling and satisfying yet have fewer than 10 calories each – perfect if you are trying to be more mindful of your weight.

Egg-filled Mushrooms on Toast

25 g (1 oz) butter

4 eggs, beaten

½ tablespoon chopped chives

1 tablespoon olive oil

4 portobello mushrooms

2 tomatoes, chopped

2 spring onions, thinly sliced

4 slices of wholemeal or sourdough bread, toasted

salt and pepper

Melt the butter in a small frying pan. Pour in the eggs and chives, season with salt and pepper and cook for 4–5 minutes, stirring occasionally, until cooked.

Meanwhile, heat the oil in a frying pan and cook the mushrooms for 3–4 minutes on each side.

Mix together the tomatoes and spring onions.

Place the toast on 4 warmed plates and top with the mushrooms, then drizzle over any pan juices.

Spoon the scrambled egg into the mushrooms and serve sprinkled with the tomato and spring onion mixture.

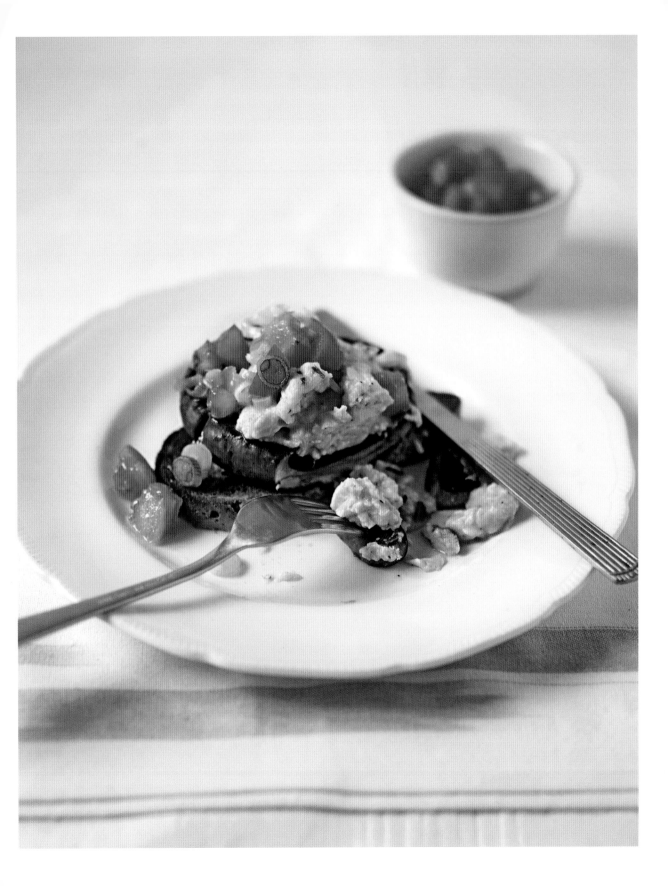

Feta, Herb & Rocket Frittata

4 eggs, beaten

2 tablespoons chopped herbs, such as chives, chervil and parsley

1 tablespoon double cream

1 tablespoon olive oil

1 small red onion, finely sliced

½ red pepper, cored, deseeded and finely sliced

100 g (3½ oz) feta cheese

handful of rocket leaves

salt and pepper

Beat the eggs, herbs and cream together in a bowl, and season with salt and pepper.

Heat the oil in a nonstick frying pan with a flameproof handle, add the onion and red pepper and cook over a medium heat for 3–4 minutes until just softened.

Pour in the egg mixture and cook for about 3 minutes until almost set, then crumble over the feta.

Place the pan under a preheated hot grill and cook for 2–3 minutes until the top of the tortilla is golden brown. Top with the rocket and serve.

- **FOR POTATO & GOATS' CHEESE FRITTATA**

Beat the eggs, herbs and cream together, then season as above. Add 150 g (5 oz) cooked and sliced new potatoes to the egg mixture and cook as above. Arrange 4 slices of firm goats' cheese over the frittata and finish cooking under a preheated high grill. Serve with a large handful of rocket leaves.

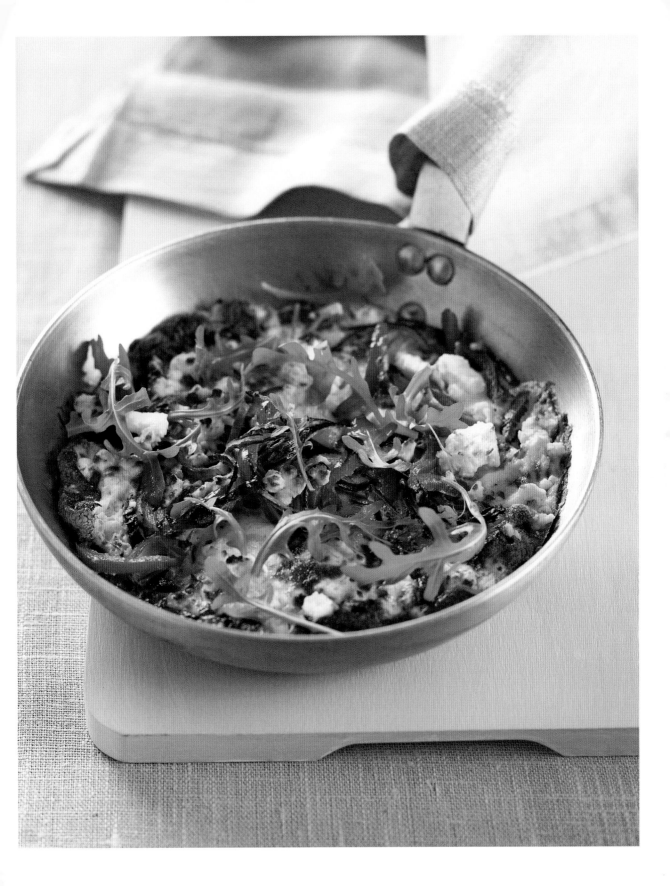

- **MAKES: 8**
- **PREPARATION TIME: 10 MINUTES**
- **COOKING TIME: 20–25 MINUTES**

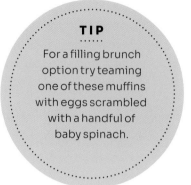

TIP

For a filling brunch option try teaming one of these muffins with eggs scrambled with a handful of baby spinach.

Cheese, Tomato & Basil Muffins

spray oil, for greasing

150 g (5 oz) wholemeal self-raising flour

½ teaspoon salt

100 g (3½ oz) fine cornmeal

65 g (2½ oz) Cheddar cheese, grated

50 g (2 oz) drained sun-dried tomatoes in oil, chopped

2 tablespoons chopped basil

1 egg, lightly beaten

300 ml (½ pint) milk

2 tablespoons extra virgin olive oil

butter, to serve

Lightly grease 8 muffin tin holes with spray oil. Sift the flour and salt into a bowl and stir in the cornmeal, 50 g (2 oz) of the cheese, the tomatoes and basil. Make a well in the centre.

Beat the egg, milk and oil together in a separate bowl or jug, pour into the well and stir together until just combined. The batter should remain a little lumpy.

Divide the batter between the prepared muffin holes and scatter over the remaining cheese. Bake in a preheated oven, 180°C (350°F), Gas Mark 4, for 20–25 minutes until risen and golden. Leave to cool in the tin for 5 minutes, then transfer to a wire rack. Serve warm with butter.

- **FOR OLIVE & PINE NUT MUFFINS**

Replace the sun-dried tomatoes with 100 g (3½ oz) chopped pitted black olives and stir in 50 g (2 oz) pine nuts. Keep the basil or use chopped fresh thyme instead. Continue the recipe as above.

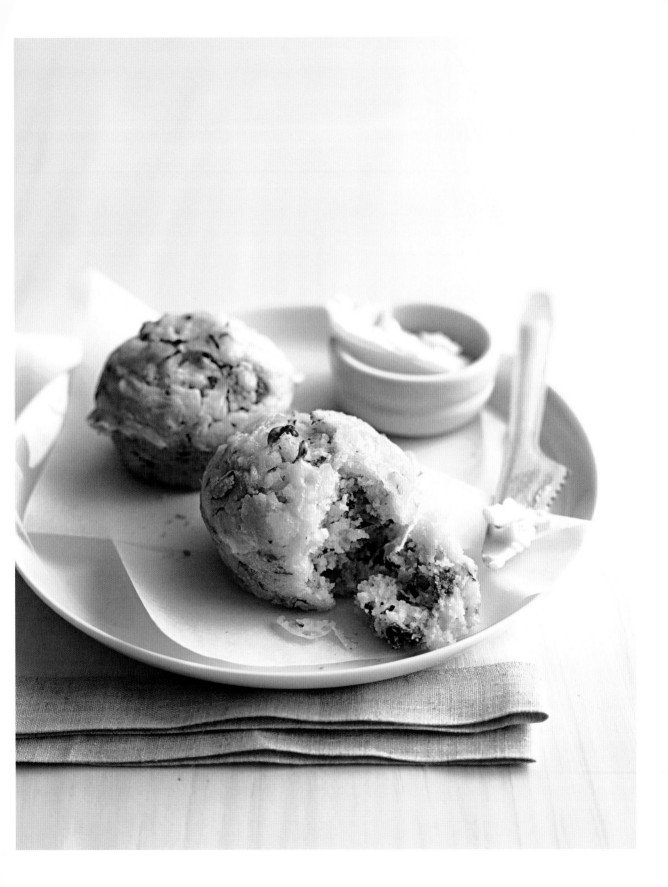

- **MAKES: 15–20**
- **PREPARATION TIME: 10 MINUTES, PLUS CHILLING**
- **COOKING TIME: 20 MINUTES**

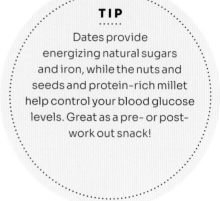

TIP

Dates provide energizing natural sugars and iron, while the nuts and seeds and protein-rich millet help control your blood glucose levels. Great as a pre- or post-work out snack!

Lemon, Pistachio & Fruit Squares

butter, for greasing

grated rind of 1 lemon

75 g (3 oz) ready-to-eat dried dates, chopped

75 g (3 oz) unsalted pistachio nuts, chopped

75 g (3 oz) flaked almonds, chopped

150 g (5 oz) millet flakes

40 g (1½ oz) cornflakes, lightly crushed

400 g (13 oz) can condensed milk

25 g (1 oz) mixed pumpkin and sunflower seeds

Grease a 28 x 18 cm (11 x 7 inch) baking tin.

Mix together all the ingredients in a large bowl until well combined and spoon the mixture into the prepared tin.

Place in a preheated oven, 180°C (350°F), Gas Mark 4, for 20 minutes.

Remove from the oven and leave the squares to cool in the tin. Mark into 15–20 squares and chill until firm. Store in an airtight container and eat within 3–5 days.

- **FOR CHOCOLATE FRUIT & NUT SQUARES**

Place 75 g (3 oz) white chocolate and 75 g (3 oz) plain dark chocolate in separate heatproof bowls over saucepans of simmering water and leave until melted. Drizzle the chocolate over the cooked and cooled squares and leave to set.

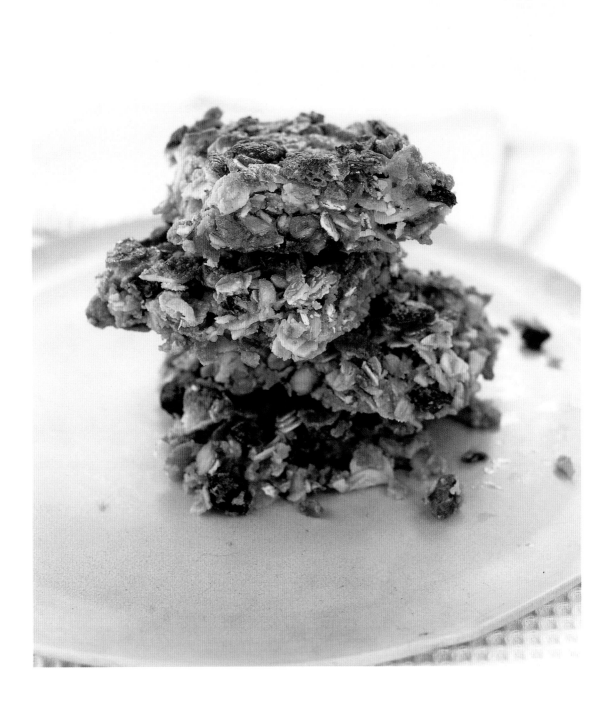

Salads & Leafy Greens

- **SERVES: 2**
- **PREPARATION TIME: 10 MINUTES**
- **COOKING TIME: 20 MINUTES**

Roast Mushroom Salad

....

4 portobello mushrooms

3 tablespoons olive oil

1 tablespoon balsamic vinegar

60 g (2 ¼ oz) coarse breadcrumbs

3 sprigs of thyme, chopped

20 g (¾ oz) mixed rocket, watercress and spinach leaves

salt and pepper

Dressing

100 g (3 ½ oz) soft goats' cheese

2 tablespoons olive oil

2 tablespoons milk

Put the mushrooms in a roasting tin and drizzle over 1 tablespoon of the olive oil and the balsamic vinegar. Cook in a preheated oven, 180°C (350°F), Gas Mark 4, for 20 minutes.

Meanwhile, spread the breadcrumbs on a baking sheet with the thyme. Pour over the remaining oil and season with salt and pepper. Place in the oven and cook for 6–8 minutes until golden and crispy.

Make the dressing. Put the cheese, oil and milk in a small saucepan and whisk over a gentle heat until the mixture reaches a pouring consistency, adding a little more milk if it is too thick.

Transfer the mushrooms to serving plates and top with the breadcrumbs. Arrange a handful of the mixed leaves to the side and drizzle with the warm dressing. Serve immediately.

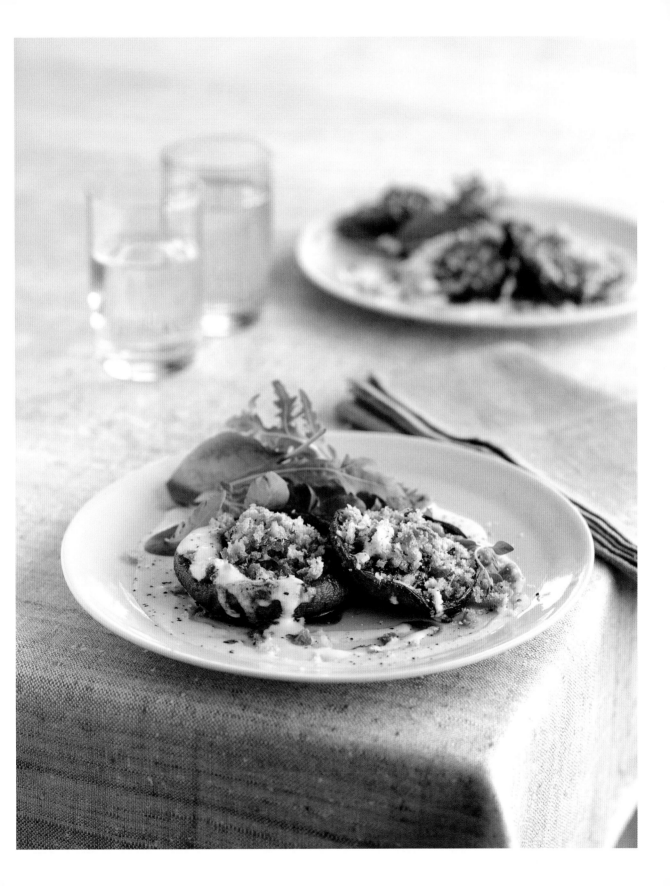

- **SERVES: 4**
- **PREPARATION TIME: 15 MINUTES**
- **COOKING TIME: 20 MINUTES**

TIP

Buckwheat is a super grain, rich in magnesium, iron and fibre which help fight fatigue and improve gut health.

Buckwheat & Salmon Salad

300 g (10 oz) buckwheat

250 g (8 oz) broccoli florets

250 g (8 oz) cherry tomatoes, halved

250 g (8 oz) smoked salmon

small bunch of parsley, chopped

4 tablespoons chopped dill

salt and pepper

Dressing

juice of 1 lemon

3 tablespoons olive oil

Put the buckwheat in a saucepan, cover with cold water and add a pinch of salt. Bring to the boil and cook for 10–15 minutes until tender but still firm and not mushy. Drain under running cold water and remove the foam that accumulates. Drain again when cool.

Bring a large saucepan of lightly salted water to the boil and blanch the broccoli florets for 2–3 minutes. Refresh in cold water and drain.

Mix the cherry tomatoes with the buckwheat and broccoli in a large salad bowl. Slice the smoked salmon and add it to the bowl with the parsley and half of the dill.

Make the dressing by whisking the lemon juice and oil. Pour the dressing over the salad, mix lightly to combine and season to taste with salt and pepper. Serve immediately, garnished with the remaining dill.

- **FOR SMOKED SALMON & SPRING GREEN SALAD**

Blanch and refresh 400 g (13 oz) assorted green vegetables, including sugar snap peas, mangetout, asparagus, green beans and peas. Put the vegetables in a large salad bowl and add 250 g (8 oz) finely sliced smoked salmon, 1 finely diced red onion, 2 tablespoons chopped parsley, 60 g (2 ¼ oz) watercress and 2 tablespoons olive oil. Season to taste with salt and pepper and mix lightly. In a small bowl make a lemon crème fraîche dressing by whisking together 4 tablespoons crème fraîche, the rind and juice of 1 lemon, 2 tablespoons chopped dill, 2 tablespoons olive oil and salt and pepper. Drizzle the dressing over the salad and serve.

- **SERVES 4**
- **PREPARATION TIME: 15 MINUTES**
- **COOKING TIME: 10 MINUTES**

Bang Bang Chicken Salad

50 g (2 oz) dried vermicelli noodles

¼ Savoy cabbage, finely shredded

1 carrot, finely chopped

½ cucumber, finely chopped

juice of 1 lime

100 g (3½ oz) peanut butter

3 tablespoons sweet chilli sauce

1 tablespoon soy sauce

1 teaspoon Chinese vinegar

2 tablespoons sesame oil

2 tablespoons vegetable oil

3 poached chicken breasts, each about 150 g (5 oz)

3 finely sliced spring onions, to garnish

Bring a large saucepan of water to the boil and cook the noodles for 2 minutes. Refresh in cold water, drain and transfer to a large salad bowl.

Add the cabbage, carrot, cucumber and lime juice to the noodles.

Gently warm the peanut butter in a small saucepan. Add the sweet chilli sauce, soy sauce, vinegar and sesame and vegetable oils and whisk to a pouring consistency. (If necessary, add a little warm water to achieve the correct consistency.) Set the sauce aside to cool slightly.

Shred the chicken breasts, add the meat to the noodle mix and combine well. Arrange on serving plates, spoon over the peanut sauce and garnish with finely sliced spring onions.

- **SERVES: 2**
- **PREPARATION TIME: 10 MINUTES**
- **COOKING TIME: 2–4 MINUTES**

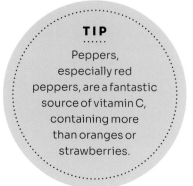

TIP

Peppers, especially red peppers, are a fantastic source of vitamin C, containing more than oranges or strawberries.

Hot Haloumi with Fattoush Salad

2 teaspoons olive oil

250 g (8 oz) haloumi cheese, thickly sliced

lemon wedges, to serve

Fattoush salad

75 g (3 oz) red pepper, cored, deseeded and finely sliced

75 g (3 oz) yellow pepper, cored, deseeded and finely sliced

75 g (3 oz) cucumber, chopped

75 g (3 oz) spring onions, finely chopped

2 tablespoons chopped flat leaf parsley

2 tablespoons chopped mint

2 tablespoons chopped coriander

Dressing

1 teaspoon crushed garlic

2 tablespoons olive oil or flaxseed oil

4 tablespoons lemon juice

salt and pepper

Heat the oil in a nonstick frying pan, add the haloumi and cook over a medium–high heat for 1–2 minutes on each side until golden brown. Remove from the pan and keep warm.

Place the peppers, cucumber, spring onions and herbs in a bowl and stir to combine.

Make the dressing. Mix the garlic with the oil and lemon juice and season to taste with salt and pepper.

Pour the dressing over the salad and toss lightly to mix. Serve with the warm haloumi and lemon wedges for squeezing over.

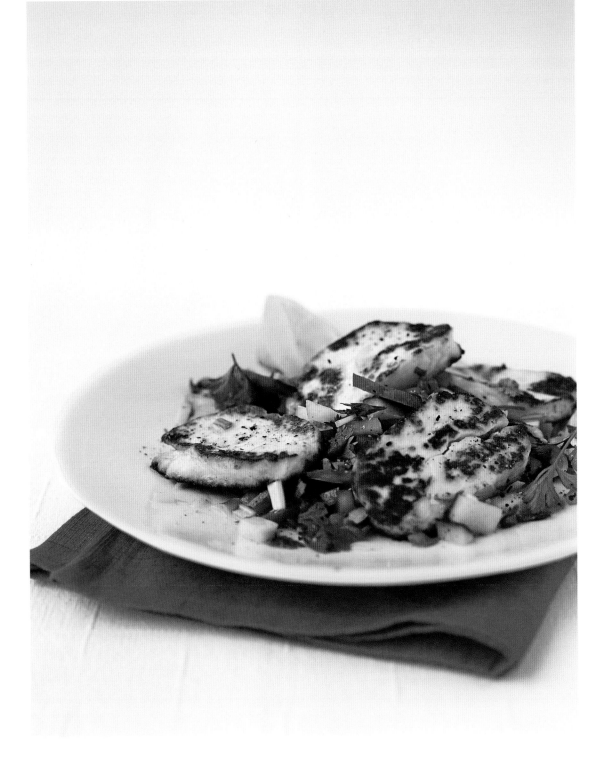

- **SERVES: 4–6**
- **PREPARATION TIME: 5 MINUTES**

Green Salad

....

400 g (13 oz) mixed baby leaves and herbs, such as watercress, frisée (curly-leaved endive), rocket, tatsoi or spinach, chives, parsley and chervil

Dressing

1 teaspoon Dijon mustard

2 tablespoons chardonnay vinegar

4 tablespoons olive oil

salt and pepper

Make the dressing by whisking together the mustard, vinegar and oil. Season to taste with salt and pepper.

Put the mixed leaves into a large salad bowl. Carefully toss the leaves and herbs with the dressing to combine and serve immediately.

....

- **FOR GREEN SALAD WITH CRUSTED GOATS' CHEESE**

Mix together 75 g (3 oz) breadcrumbs, 20 g (¾ oz) crushed hazelnuts, 2 tablespoons chopped parsley and 1 crushed garlic clove. Season to taste with salt and pepper. Cut 100 g (3½ oz) goats' cheese into rounds, dip them in flour, then in lightly beaten egg, then in the breadcrumb mixture. Heat 2 tablespoons vegetable oil in a large frying pan over a medium heat and fry the cheese slices for 3 minutes on each side until golden and crispy. Drain on kitchen paper and serve with the green salad as above.

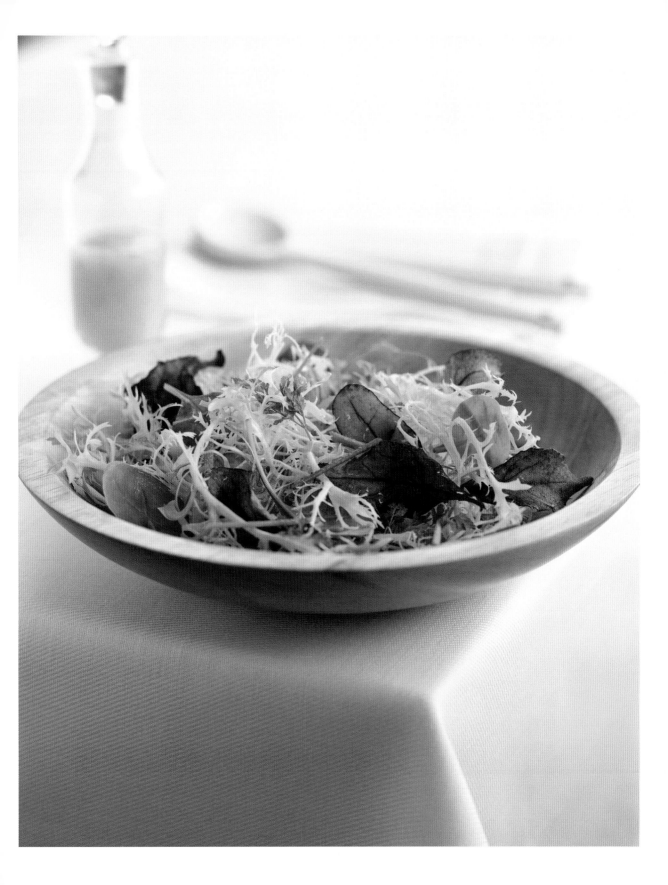

- **SERVES: 4**
- **PREPARATION TIME: 15 MINUTES**
- **COOKING TIME: 45–50 MINUTES**

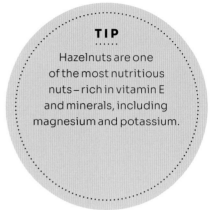

TIP

Hazelnuts are one of the most nutritious nuts – rich in vitamin E and minerals, including magnesium and potassium.

Roasted Summer Vegetables

1 red pepper, cored, deseeded and thickly sliced

1 yellow pepper, cored, deseeded and thickly sliced

1 aubergine, cut into chunks

2 yellow or green courgettes, cut into chunks

1 red onion, cut into wedges

6 garlic cloves

2 tablespoons extra virgin rapeseed oil or olive oil

150 g (5 oz) yellow and red baby plum tomatoes

4–5 sprigs of thyme

150 g (5 oz) hazelnuts

125 g (4 oz) rocket leaves

2 tablespoons raspberry or balsamic vinegar

salt and pepper

handful of mustard cress, to garnish (optional)

Toss all the vegetables, except the tomatoes, in a large bowl with the oil. Season with a little salt and pepper and add the thyme. Tip into a large roasting tin and place in a preheated oven, 190°C (375°F), Gas Mark 5, for 40–45 minutes or until the vegetables are tender. Add the tomatoes and return to the oven for a further 5 minutes or until the tomatoes are just softened and beginning to burst.

Meanwhile, tip the hazelnuts into a small roasting tin and place in the oven for about 10–12 minutes or until golden and the skin is peeling away. Leave to cool, then remove the excess skin and crush lightly.

Toss the rocket leaves gently with the mixed, roasted vegetables and heap on to large plates. Scatter over the crushed hazelnuts and drizzle with the vinegar. Scatter over the mustard cress, if using, and serve immediately.

- **FOR ROASTED VEGETABLE PASTA SAUCE**

Roast the vegetables as above, then tip into a large saucepan with the tomatoes, 500 ml (17 fl oz) passata and 150 ml (¼ pint) vegetable stock. Bring to the boil, then reduce the heat and simmer gently for 20 minutes. Remove from the heat and use a hand-held blender to blend until smooth. Season with salt and pepper, to taste, and serve with bowls of hot pasta. Alternatively, stir in an extra 250 ml (8 fl oz) vegetable stock to make soup.

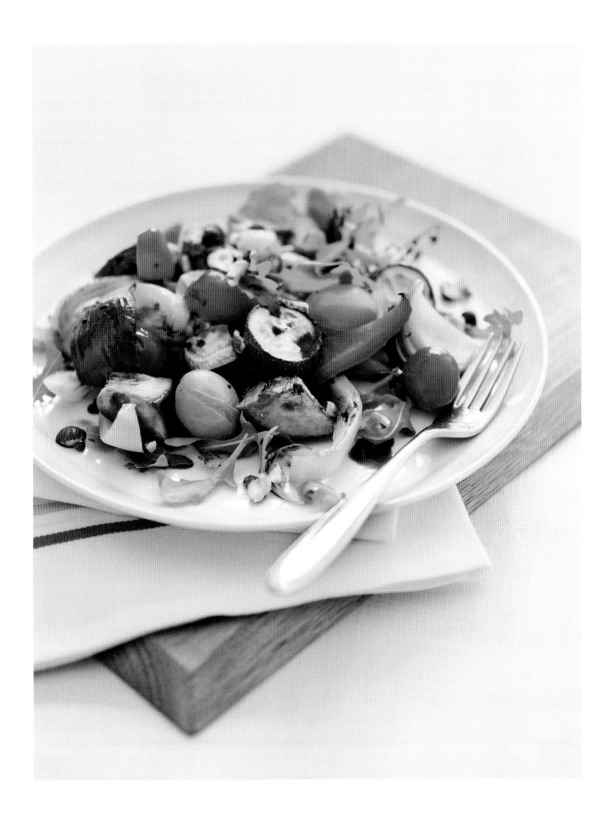

- **SERVES: 4–6**
- **PREPARATION TIME: 10 MINUTES, PLUS COOLING**
- **COOKING TIME: 2–3 MINUTES**

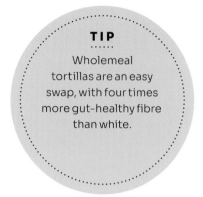

TIP

Wholemeal tortillas are an easy swap, with four times more gut-healthy fibre than white.

Healthy Bread Salad

2 wholemeal flatbreads or flour tortillas

1 large green pepper, cored, deseeded and diced

1 Lebanese cucumber, diced

250 g (8 oz) cherry tomatoes, halved

½ red onion, finely chopped

2 tablespoons chopped mint

2 tablespoons chopped parsley

2 tablespoons chopped coriander

3 tablespoons olive oil

juice of 1 lemon

salt and pepper

Toast the flatbreads or tortillas on a preheated ridged griddle pan or under a preheated hot grill for 2–3 minutes or until charred. Leave to cool, then tear into bite-sized pieces.

Put the green pepper, cucumber, tomatoes, onion and herbs in a serving bowl, add the oil and lemon juice and season with salt and pepper, tossing well. Add the bread and stir again. Serve immediately.

- **FOR TOMATO & BREAD SALAD**

Chop 750 g (1½ lb) tomatoes and put into a large bowl. Add 4 slices of diced day-old bread, 1 bunch of basil leaves, 125 g (4 oz) pitted black olives, 75 ml (3 fl oz) olive oil, 1 tablespoon balsamic vinegar and salt and pepper. Toss well and serve.

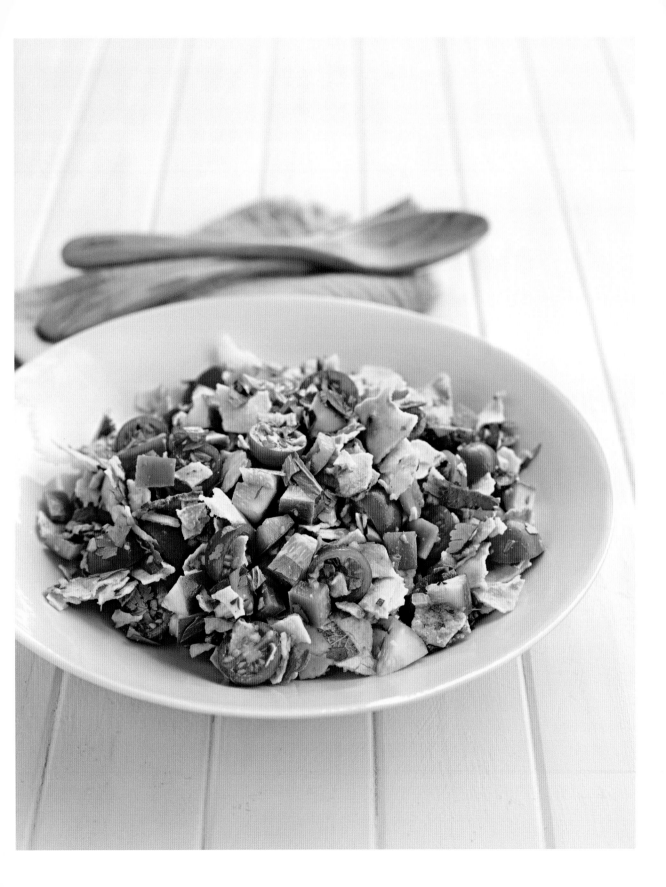

- **SERVES: 4**
- **PREPARATION TIME: 15 MINUTES**
- **COOKING TIME: 2–3 MINUTES**

Chicken & Aduki Bean Salad

1 green pepper, cored, deseeded and chopped

1 red pepper, cored, deseeded and chopped

1 small red onion, finely chopped

400 g (13 oz) can aduki beans, drained

200 g (7 oz) can sweetcorn, drained

small bunch of coriander, chopped

50 g (2 oz) unsweetened coconut chips or flakes

250 g (8 oz) cooked chicken breast, shredded

small handful of alfalfa shoots (optional)

Dressing

3 tablespoons light groundnut oil

2 tablespoons light soy sauce

2 teaspoons peeled and grated fresh root ginger

1 tablespoon rice vinegar

Mix together the green and red peppers, onion, aduki beans, sweetcorn and half the coriander in a large bowl. Whisk together the dressing ingredients in a separate bowl, then stir 3 tablespoons into the bean salad. Spoon the salad into serving dishes.

Place the coconut chips or flakes in a nonstick frying pan over a medium heat and dry-fry for 2–3 minutes or until lightly golden brown, stirring continuously.

Scatter the shredded chicken and remaining coriander leaves over the bean salad and sprinkle with the toasted coconut and alfalfa shoots, if using. Serve with the remaining dressing.

- **FOR PRAWN, AVOCADO & COCONUT SALAD**

Make as above, replacing the chicken with 250 g (8 oz) cooked, peeled prawns. Dice the flesh of 1 firm, ripe avocado, toss in 1 tablespoon of lime juice and add to the bean salad. Serve as above.

- **SERVES: 4–6**
- **PREPARATION TIME: 10 MINUTES, PLUS COOLING**
- **COOKING TIME: 15 MINUTES**

TIP

Cooking potatoes and then serving them cold has the advantage of decreasing their glycaemic value, meaning they produce a steadier rise in blood glucose.

Potato Salad

1 kg (2 lb) new potatoes

50 g (2 oz) blue cheese

2 tablespoons soured cream

1 tablespoon lemon juice

175 ml (6 fl oz) mayonnaise

2 tablespoons chopped parsley

40 g (1½ oz) toasted walnuts

salt and pepper

Halve the potatoes and cook in lightly salted boiling water until tender. Rinse under cold water and leave to cool.

Place the blue cheese, soured cream, lemon juice and mayonnaise in a bowl and combine well.

Add the potatoes, and mix the dressing through the cooked potatoes together with the chopped parsley.

Garnish with the toasted walnuts, season to taste with salt and pepper, and serve.

- **SERVES: 4**
- **PREPARATION TIME: 10 MINUTES**
- **COOKING TIME: ABOUT 1 HOUR 10 MINUTES**

TIP

Beetroot is a natural source of nitrates which can lower blood pressure and improve blood flow.

Roasted Beetroot & Bean Salad

1 kg (2 lb) raw beetroot, peeled

1½ tablespoons extra virgin rapeseed oil, plus extra to serve

2 teaspoons cumin seeds

4 tablespoons balsamic vinegar

250 g (8 oz) green beans, trimmed

1 red onion, thinly sliced

250 g (8 oz) ricotta cheese

finely grated rind of 1 lemon

small bunch of basil, chopped, a few leaves reserved for garnish

1 multigrain or cereal baguette, sliced

1 tablespoon balsamic glaze

salt and pepper

Cut the beetroot into wedges or in half, if small. Toss with the oil and cumin seeds and season with salt and pepper. Tip into a roasting tin and place in a preheated oven, 180°C (350°F), Gas Mark 4, for 45 minutes. Pour over the balsamic vinegar and toss to coat. Return to the oven for a further 20 minutes or until the beetroot is tender and slightly sticky.

Cook the beans in a large saucepan of lightly salted boiling water for 2–3 minutes or until just tender. Drain and toss with the beetroot and onion in a bowl.

Mix together in a bowl the ricotta, lemon rind and basil and season with salt and pepper. Spread over the baguette slices, place on a grill pan and cook under a preheated medium-hot grill for 3 minutes or until hot and lightly golden.

Heap the beetroot and bean salad into bowls and top with the ricotta croutons. Drizzle with a little balsamic glaze and extra virgin rapeseed oil and scatter with the extra basil leaves. Serve immediately.

- **FOR WINTERY ROAST PARSNIP & CARROT SALAD**

Mix together 500 g (1 lb) parsnips and 500 g (1 lb) carrots, both cut into batons, with the oil, cumin seeds and 3–4 thyme sprigs in a roasting tin. Place in the preheated oven for about 30 minutes or until tender. Spoon into a serving dish and drizzle over 2 tablespoons runny honey mixed with 1 tablespoon balsamic vinegar. Make the croutons as above, replacing the basil with 1 bunch of thyme. Serve the roast vegetables with salad leaves, scattered with 2 tablespoons toasted hazelnuts, if liked.

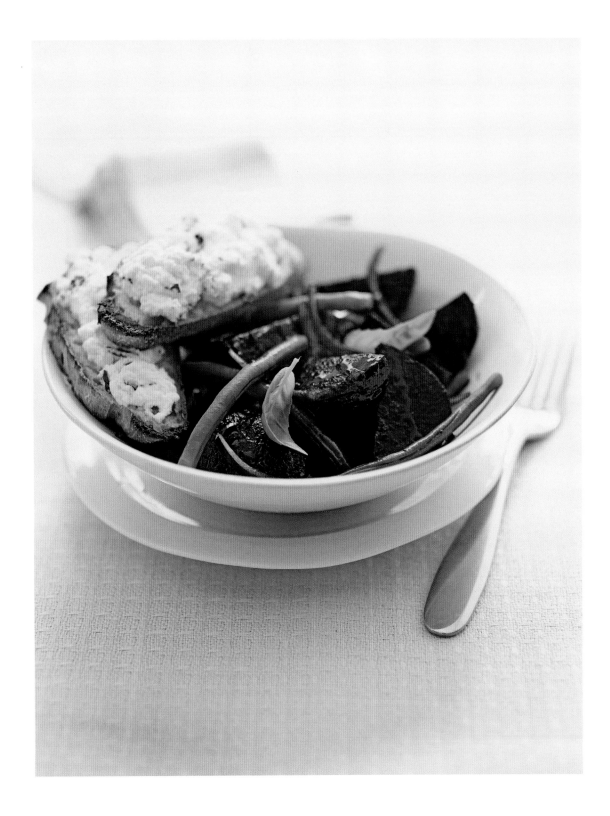

- **SERVES: 4**
- **PREPARATION TIME: 15 MINUTES, PLUS COOLING**
- **COOKING TIME: 10–12 MINUTES**

TIP

Red-skinned apples have higher amounts of cortisol-friendly flavanols and other anti-inflammatory phytochemcials than green apples.

Apple, Blue Cheese & Nut Salad

15 g (½ oz) unsalted butter

2 tablespoons caster sugar

2 red dessert apples, cored and cut into thin wedges

75 g (3 oz) walnut pieces

½ small red cabbage, thinly sliced

2 celery sticks, chopped

150 g (5 oz) blue cheese, such as dolcelatte, crumbled

Dressing

2 tablespoons walnut oil

2 tablespoons olive oil

2 tablespoons balsamic vinegar

salt and pepper

Melt the butter in a frying pan, add the sugar and stir over a low heat until the sugar has dissolved.

Add the apples to the pan and cook for 3–4 minutes on each side until they start to caramelize, then stir in the walnuts and cook for 1 minute. Remove from the heat and leave to cool.

Place the red cabbage and celery in a bowl, then add the cooled apple and walnut mixture.

Make the dressing. Place the oils and vinegar in a screw-top jar with salt and pepper to taste, add the lid and shake well.

Drizzle the dressing over the ingredients in the bowl and toss together. Serve immediately, scattered with the blue cheese.

- **FOR PEAR, SPINACH & STILTON SALAD**

Melt the butter and heat the sugar until dissolved as above. Add 2 cored and thinly sliced firm but ripe pears in place of the apples and cook until caramelized, then stir in the walnuts as above. Place 200 g (7 oz) baby spinach leaves in a bowl, instead of the red cabbage and celery, and add the pear and walnut mixture. Prepare the dressing as above, add to the bowl and gently coat the salad ingredients in the dressing. Divide between 4 plates, scatter with 150 g (5 oz) crumbled Stilton and serve immediately.

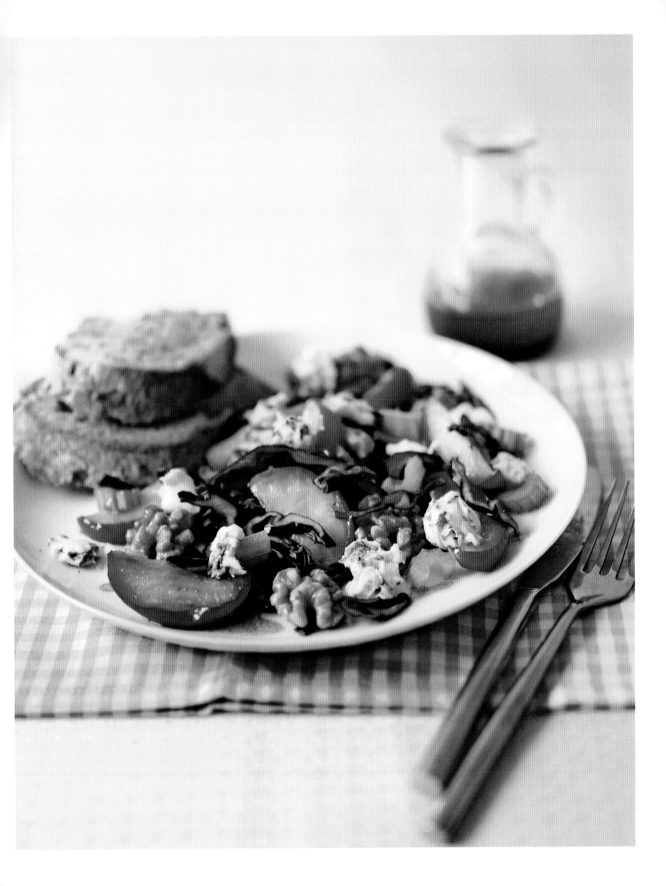

- **SERVES: 4–6**
- **PREPARATION TIME: 10 MINUTES**
- **COOKING TIME: 10 MINUTES**

Courgette, Feta & Mint Salad

3 green courgettes

2 yellow courgettes

olive oil

small bunch of mint

40 g (1½ oz) feta cheese

salt and pepper

Dressing

2 tablespoons olive oil

grated rind and juice of 1 lemon

Slice the courgettes thinly lengthways into long ribbons. Drizzle with oil and season with salt and pepper. Heat a griddle pan to very hot and grill the courgettes in batches until marked by the griddle on both sides, then place in a large salad bowl.

Make the dressing by whisking together the oil and the grated lemon rind and juice. Season to taste with salt and pepper.

Roughly chop the mint, reserving some leaves for garnish. Carefully mix together the courgettes, mint and dressing. Transfer them to a large salad bowl, then crumble the feta over the top, garnish with the remaining mint leaves and serve.

- **FOR MARINATED COURGETTE SALAD**

Thinly slice 3 courgettes lengthways and put them in a non-metallic bowl with ½ deseeded and sliced red chilli, 4 tablespoons lemon juice, 1 crushed garlic clove and 4 tablespoons olive oil. Season to taste with salt and pepper. Leave the salad to marinate, covered, for at least 1 hour. Roughly chop a small bunch of mint, toss with the salad and serve immediately.

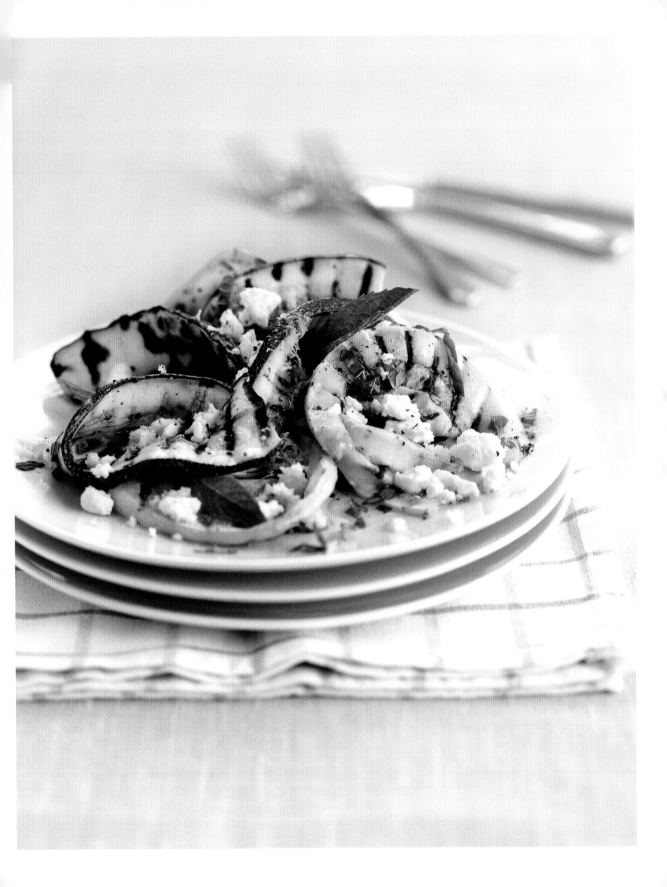

- **SERVES: 4**
- **PREPARATION TIME: 20 MINUTES**

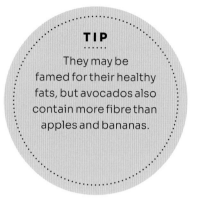

TIP

They may be famed for their healthy fats, but avocados also contain more fibre than apples and bananas.

Chicken & Avocado Salad

375 g (12 oz) cold cooked chicken

1 large avocado

1 punnet of mustard and cress

150 g (5 oz) mixed salad leaves

50 g (2 oz) mixed toasted seeds, such as pumpkin and sunflower

toasted wholegrain rye bread or flatbreads, to serve

Dressing

2 tablespoons apple juice

2 tablespoons natural yogurt

1 teaspoon clear honey

1 teaspoon wholegrain mustard

salt and pepper

Thinly slice the chicken. Peel and stone the avocado, cut it into wedges then mix it with the mustard and cress and salad leaves in a large bowl. Add the chicken and toasted seeds and stir to combine.

Make the dressing by whisking together the apple juice, yogurt, honey and mustard. Season to taste with salt and pepper.

Pour the dressing over the salad and toss to coat. Serve the salad with toasted wholegrain rye bread or rolled up in flatbreads.

- **FOR CRAB, APPLE & AVOCADO SALAD**

Prepare the salad in the same way, using 300 g (10 oz) cooked, fresh white crab meat instead of the chicken. Cut 1 apple into thin matchsticks and toss with a little lemon juice to stop it from discolouring, then add it to the salad. Make a dressing by whisking 2 tablespoons apple juice with 3 tablespoons olive oil, a squeeze of lemon juice and 1 finely diced shallot. Season to taste with salt and pepper. Pour the dressing over the salad, stir carefully to mix and serve.

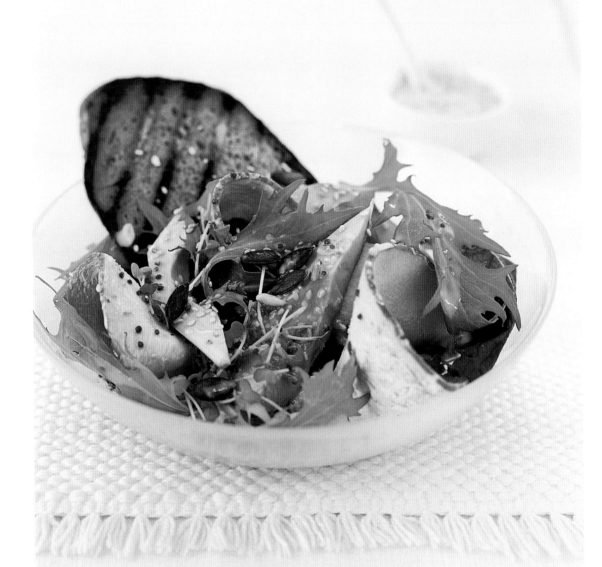

- **SERVES: 4**
- **PREPARATION TIME: 10 MINUTES**
- **COOKING TIME: 3 MINUTES**

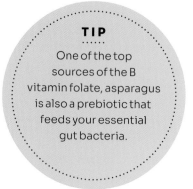

TIP

One of the top sources of the B vitamin folate, asparagus is also a prebiotic that feeds your essential gut bacteria.

Spring Vegetable Salad

200 g (7 oz) fresh or frozen peas

200 g (7 oz) asparagus, trimmed

200 g (7 oz) sugar snap peas

2 courgettes

1 fennel bulb

Dressing

grated rind and juice of 1 lemon

1 teaspoon Dijon mustard

1 teaspoon clear honey

1 tablespoon chopped flat leaf parsley

1 tablespoon olive oil

Put the peas, asparagus and sugar snap peas in a saucepan of salted boiling water and simmer for 3 minutes. Drain, then refresh under cold running water.

Cut the courgettes into long, thin ribbons and thinly slice the fennel. Transfer all the vegetables to a large salad bowl and mix together.

Make the dressing by whisking together the lemon rind and juice, mustard, honey, parsley and oil in another bowl. Toss the dressing through the vegetables and serve.

- **FOR SPRING VEGETABLES WITH BEETROOT DRESSING**

Prepare the vegetables as above and set aside. Finely slice ½ red onion and 1 garlic clove. Heat 2 tablespoons olive oil in a saucepan over a medium heat and gently cook the onion and garlic. Add 4 chopped precooked beetroot and 6 roughly chopped sun-blushed tomatoes and continue to cook for 3 minutes. When the onions start to colour, deglaze the pan with 2 tablespoons balsamic vinegar. Cook for 1 minute, then add 100 ml (3½ fl oz) chicken or vegetable stock. Reduce the stock by a quarter, then leave to cool. Transfer the mixture to a food processor or blender and whiz until smooth. Season with salt and pepper and add up to 2 tablespoons cream until the dressing reaches a drizzling consistency. Drizzle the dressing over the vegetables and serve.

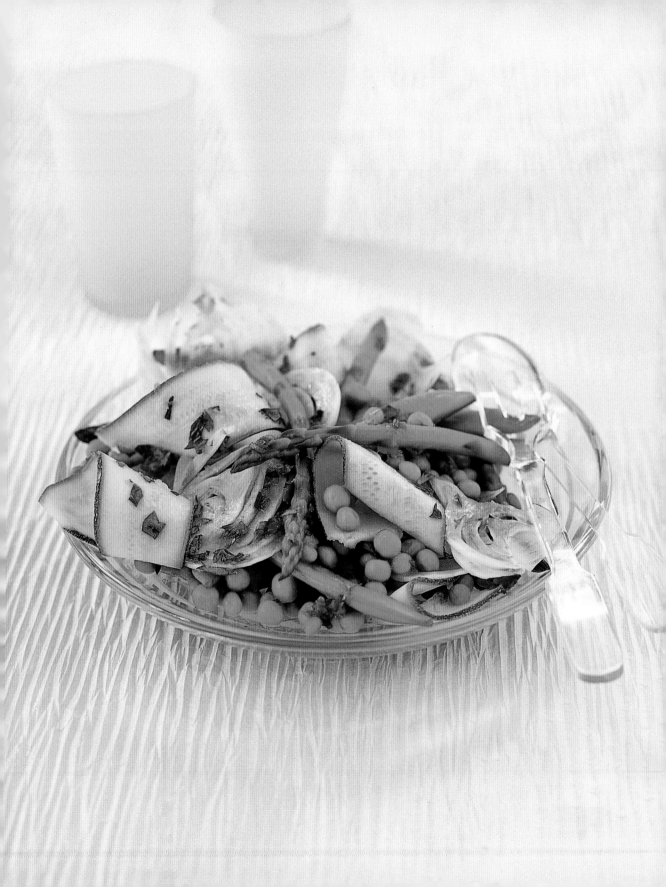

- **SERVES: 4**
- **PREPARATION TIME: 15 MINUTES**
- **COOKING TIME: 10 MINUTES**

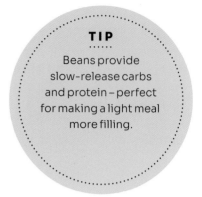

TIP

Beans provide slow-release carbs and protein – perfect for making a light meal more filling.

Pea & Broad Bean Salad

150 g (5 oz) frozen peas

150 g (5 oz) broad beans

75 g (3 oz) pea shoots

small bunch of mint, roughly chopped

150 g (5 oz) feta cheese

Dressing

1 teaspoon Dijon mustard

2 tablespoons olive oil

1 tablespoon white wine vinegar

salt and pepper

Bring a large saucepan of lightly salted water to the boil and cook the peas for 2 minutes. Refresh in cold water. Cook the broad beans for 3 minutes, refresh and peel to reveal the bright green inside. Mix the peas and broad beans with the pea shoots and roughly chopped mint.

Make the dressing by whisking the mustard, oil and vinegar. Season to taste with salt and pepper.

Crumble the feta into the salad, then carefully mix in the dressing and serve.

- **FOR PEA, BROAD BEAN & CHORIZO SALAD**

Prepare the peas and broad beans as above. Put them in a bowl with the pea shoots and add 1 grated courgette. Thinly slice 3 chorizo sausages diagonally and fry in a hot frying pan until golden and crispy. Drain on kitchen paper, then add to the salad. Whisk the dressing ingredients as above and toss the salad with the mint and feta. Serve immediately.

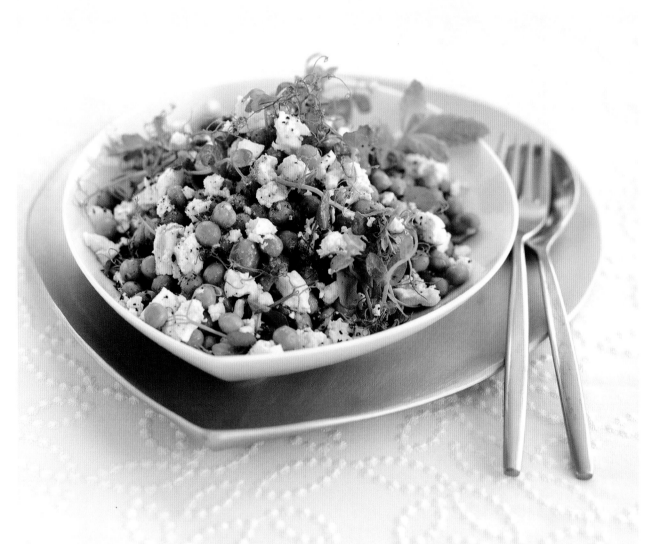

- **SERVES: 4**
- **PREPARATION TIME: 20 MINUTES**

Orange & Avocado Salad

4 large juicy oranges

2 small ripe avocados

2 teaspoons cardamom pods

3 tablespoons olive oil

1 tablespoon clear honey

pinch of allspice

2 teaspoons lemon juice

salt and pepper

sprigs of watercress, to garnish

Cut the skin and the white membrane off the oranges. Working over a bowl to catch the juice, cut between the membranes to remove the segments. Peel and stone the avocados, slice the flesh and toss gently with the orange segments. Pile on to serving plates.

Reserve a few whole cardamom pods for garnishing. Crush the remainder using a mortar and pestle to extract the seeds or place them in a small bowl and crush with the end of a rolling pin. Pick out and discard the pods.

Mix the seeds with the oil, honey, allspice and lemon juice. Season to taste with salt and pepper and stir in the reserved orange juice. Garnish the salads with sprigs of watercress and the reserved cardamom pods and serve with the dressing spooned over the top.

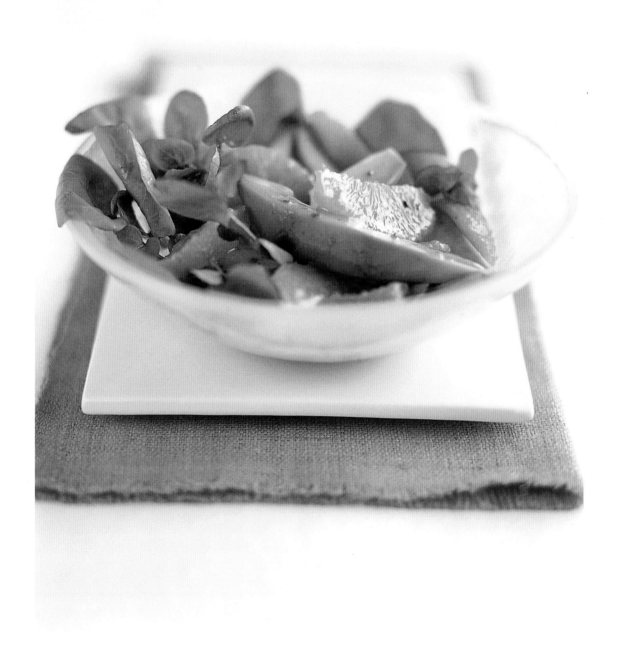

Smoked Trout & Grape Salad

....

200 g (7 oz) smoked trout

160 g (5½ oz) red seedless grapes

75 g (3 oz) watercress

1 fennel bulb

Dressing

3 tablespoons mayonnaise

4 cornichons, finely diced

1½ tablespoons capers, chopped

2 tablespoons lemon juice

salt and pepper

Flake the smoked trout into bite-sized pieces, removing any bones, and place in a large salad bowl.

Wash and drain the grapes and watercress and add them to the bowl. Finely slice the fennel and add to the mix.

Make the dressing by mixing the mayonnaise, cornichons, capers and lemon juice. Season to taste with salt and pepper, then carefully mix through the salad and serve.

....

- **FOR CRISPY TROUT SALAD**

Add 1 finely chopped hard-boiled egg, 2 finely chopped anchovy fillets and 1 tablespoon chopped parsley to the dressing. Prepare the grapes, watercress and fennel as above, adding 1 green apple, cut into matchsticks. Season 2 pieces of fresh trout, each about 140 g (4½ oz), with salt and pepper. Heat 1 tablespoon vegetable oil in a frying pan over a high heat and cook the trout, skin side down, for 4 minutes, pressing it down with a fish slice to give an evenly crispy skin. Turn over the fish and cook for a further 2 minutes or until it is just cooked through. Remove from the pan. Toss the salad with the dressing and serve immediately with the crispy trout.

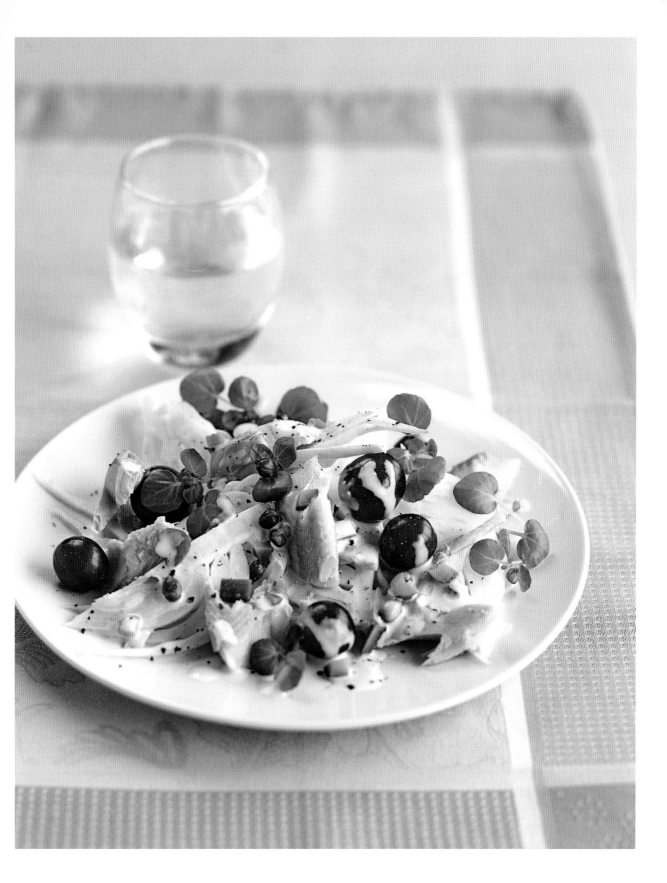

- **SERVES: 4**
- **PREPARATION TIME: 25 MINUTES**
- **COOKING TIME: 4–10 MINUTES**

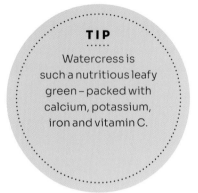

Sesame-crusted Salmon Salad

4 spring onions

2 egg whites

1 tablespoon white sesame seeds

1 tablespoon black sesame seeds

500 g (1 lb) salmon fillet

1 frisée (curly-leaved endive), divided into leaves

2 bunches of watercress

salt and pepper

Dressing

3 tablespoons white wine vinegar

5 tablespoons vegetable oil

1 tablespoon sesame oil

1 tablespoon soy sauce

1 teaspoon caster sugar

bunch of chives, finely chopped

Cut the spring onions into thin strips and put them in cold water.

Lightly beat the egg whites. Mix the white and black sesame seeds with salt and pepper on a large plate. Dip the salmon fillet in the egg whites then roll it in the sesame seeds. Pat the salmon on the seeds all over to give a good, even coating. Heat a griddle pan, add the salmon and cook for 2 minutes each side for rare or 5 minutes for well done.

Make the dressing by mixing together the vinegar, oils, soy sauce, caster sugar and chives. Toss the frisée leaves and watercress in the dressing. Arrange the leaves on a large serving dish.

Finely slice the salmon fillet and place on the dish. Drain the spring onion curls, dry them on kitchen paper and sprinkle over the salmon. Serve immediately.

- **FOR SASHIMI SALMON SALAD**

Grate 1 raw beetroot and 2 carrots and mix with 100 g (3½ oz) rocket. Make the dressing as above. Mix together 1 tablespoon each white and black sesame seeds. Slice as thinly as possible 2 skinless fillets of fresh salmon, each 150 g (5 oz), and arrange on individual plates. Drizzle the dressing over the salad, garnish with the sesame seeds and serve with the salmon.

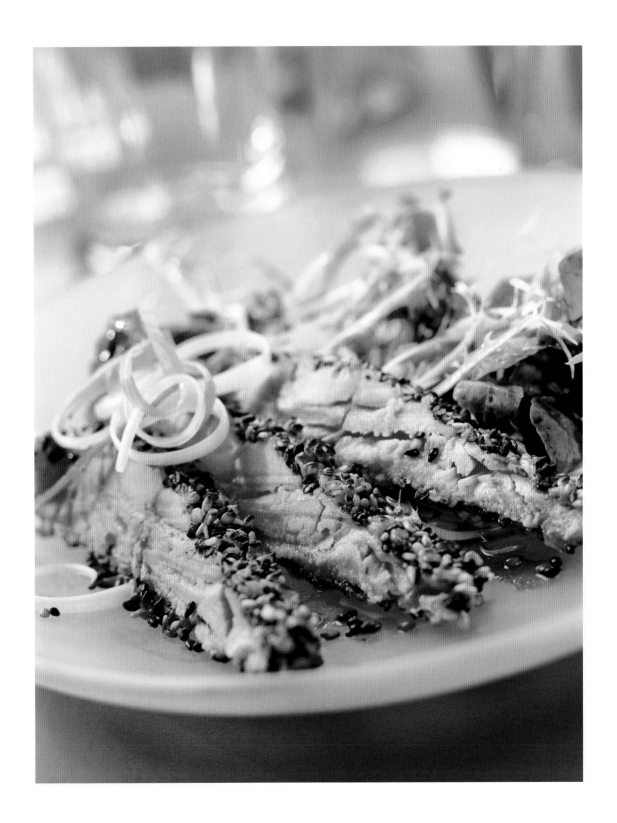

- **SERVES: 4**
- **PREPARATION TIME: 15 MINUTES**
- **COOKING TIME: 4 MINUTES**

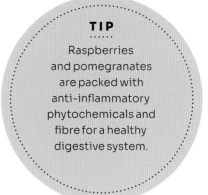

TIP

Raspberries and pomegranates are packed with anti-inflammatory phytochemicals and fibre for a healthy digestive system.

Raspberry Salad with Toasties

½ red onion, thinly sliced

125 g (4 oz) mixed salad leaves, including baby red chard leaves

100 g (3½ oz) fresh raspberries

2 tablespoons balsamic vinegar

1 pomegranate

8 slices, about 75 g (3 oz), wholemeal French bread

250 g (8 oz) cottage cheese

paprika, to garnish

Put the onion in a bowl with the salad leaves and raspberries. Drizzle over the vinegar and toss together.

Cut the pomegranate into quarters, flex the skin and pop out the seeds. Sprinkle half the seeds over the salad, then transfer the salad to 4 serving plates.

Toast the bread on both sides and arrange 2 slices in the centre of each serving plate. Spoon the cottage cheese on to the toast, sprinkle with the remaining pomegranate seeds and a little paprika and serve.

- **FOR RASPBERRY SALAD WITH RASPBERRY DRESSING**

Prepare the salad as above, but make a dressing by putting 100 g (3½ oz) raspberries, 100 ml (3½ fl oz) raspberry vinegar, 150 ml (¼ pint) olive oil, 1 teaspoon caster sugar, 1 teaspoon Dijon mustard, 2 tablespoons chopped tarragon and 1 chopped garlic clove in a food processor or blender. Whiz until smooth, then taste and adjust the seasoning with salt and pepper. If you would like the dressing really smooth pour it through a fine sieve. It will keep, covered, for up to 7 days in the refrigerator.

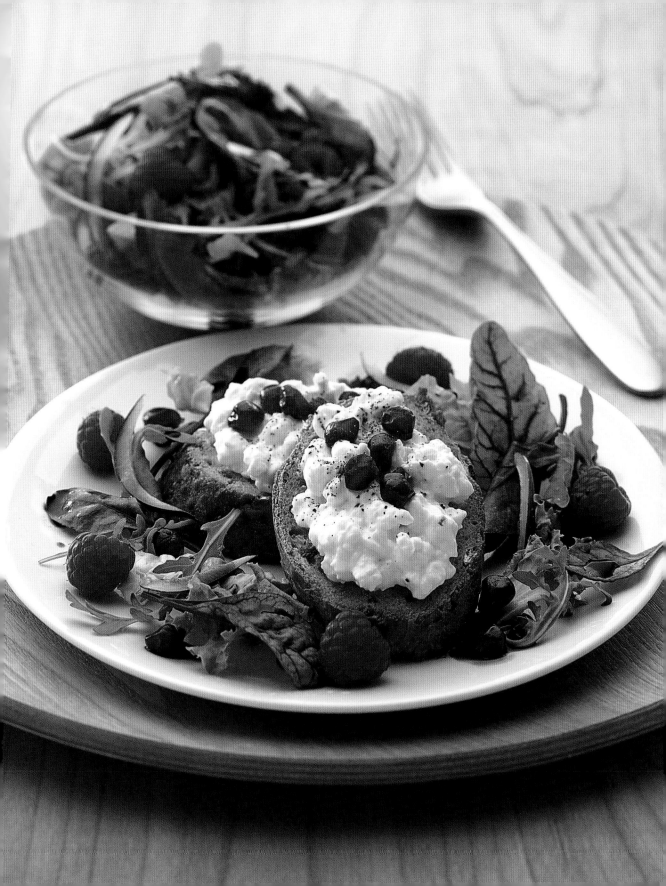

Tomato & Mozzarella Salad

....

500 g (1 lb) ripe tomatoes, preferably different types, such as heirloom, cherry and plum

about 3 tablespoons olive oil

2 tablespoons aged balsamic vinegar

small handful of basil leaves

150 g (5 oz) mini mozzarella balls

salt and pepper

Cut half the tomatoes into thick slices and the other half into wedges. Arrange the slices on a large serving plate, slightly overlapping.

Put the tomato wedges into a bowl and drizzle with olive oil and balsamic vinegar. Season to taste with salt and pepper. Mix carefully and arrange on top of the tomato slices.

Add the basil leaves and mozzarella balls to the salad. Drizzle the salad with more olive oil and balsamic vinegar, season to taste with salt and pepper and serve.

....

- **FOR TOMATO & PASTA SALAD**

Cook 250 g (8 oz) fusilli or penne until it is just tender, and drain. Chop 500 g (1 lb) tomatoes into chunks and stir through the still warm pasta, coat with olive oil and season to taste with salt and pepper. Mix through a large handful of torn basil leaves, garnish with Parmesan cheese shavings and serve.

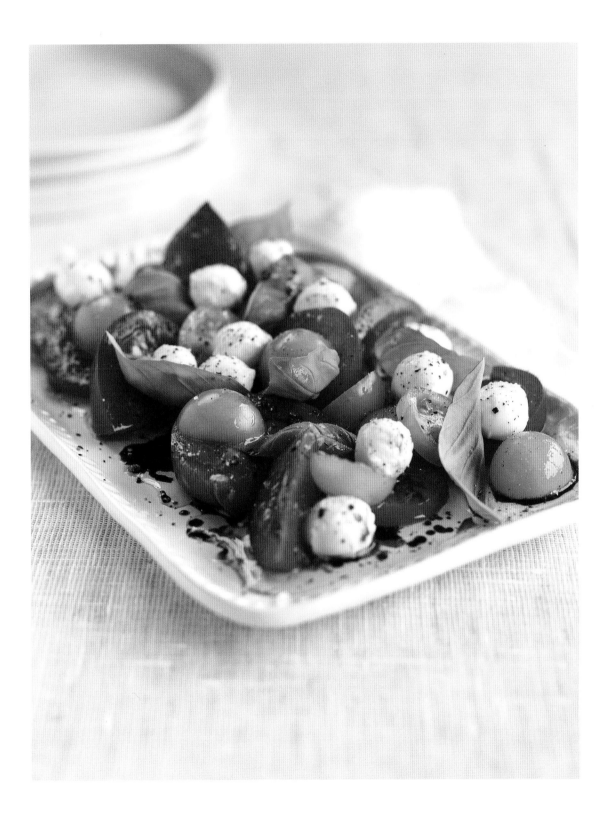

Snacks
&
Starters

- **SERVES: 6**
- **PREPARATION TIME: 5 MINUTES, PLUS MARINATING (OPTIONAL)**
- **COOKING TIME: 1 MINUTE**

Citrus Olives

....

2 teaspoons fennel seeds

finely grated rind and juice of
½ lemon

finely grated rind and juice of
¼ orange

75 ml (3 fl oz) olive oil

400 g (13 oz) mixed olives

Place the fennel seeds in a small, dry frying pan and toast for
30 seconds until they start to pop and emit an aroma. Remove
from the pan and roughly crush.

Mix together the fennel seeds, lemon and orange rind and juice and
oil in a non-metallic bowl, then stir in the olives. Serve immediately or
cover and leave to marinate overnight in a cool place before serving.

....

- **FOR CITRUS OLIVE BUTTER**

Mix together 75 g (3 oz) finely chopped pitted olives, 50 g (2 oz)
softened butter and 1 teaspoon each of grated lemon and orange
rind in a bowl, then add 1 tablespoon finely chopped parsley. Spoon
on to a sheet of clingfilm. Form into a cylinder and tightly roll up,
twisting the ends to secure, then store in the freezer or refrigerator.
Cut off slices to serve on top of baked or grilled white fish.

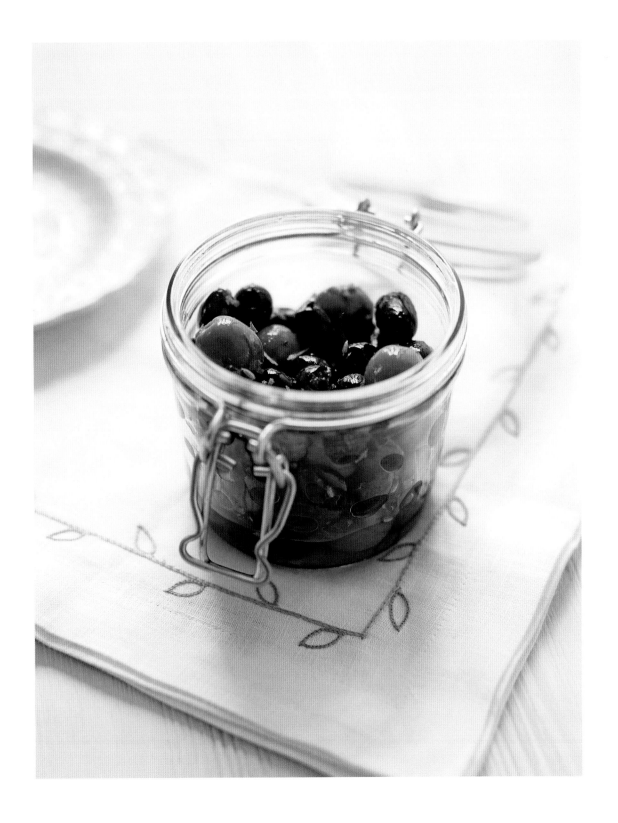

- **SERVES: 4**
- **PREPARATION TIME: 5 MINUTES**
- **COOKING TIME: 35-40 MINUTES**

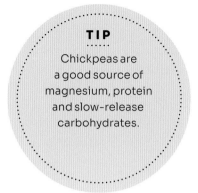

TIP

Chickpeas are a good source of magnesium, protein and slow-release carbohydrates.

Moroccan-style Spiced Chickpeas

2 x 400 g (13 oz) cans chickpeas, drained and rinsed

1 tablespoon olive oil

1 tablespoon rose harissa paste

1 tablespoon Moroccan or Middle Eastern spice mix, such as baharat

½ teaspoon salt

Dry the chickpeas on kitchen paper to remove any excess water.

Mix all the remaining ingredients together in a large bowl. Add the chickpeas and toss in the spice mix to coat.

Spread the chickpeas out in a single layer on a rimmed baking sheet and roast in a preheated oven, 200°C (400°F), Gas Mark 6, for 35-40 minutes until a deep golden colour. Leave to cool before serving.

- **FOR CURRY SPICED ROASTED MIXED NUTS**

Place 1 tablespoon sunflower oil in a small bowl and stir in 1 tablespoon medium curry powder and 1 teaspoon cumin seeds. Add 250 g (8 oz) mixed raw unsalted nuts, such as cashew nuts, macadamia nuts and almonds, and turn to coat in the spice mix. Spread out in a single layer on a nonstick baking sheet and roast in a preheated oven, 180°C (350°F), Gas Mark 4, for 10 minutes, shaking once, until lightly golden. Remove from the oven, sprinkle with 1 teaspoon sea salt and leave to cool. Serve in bowls as a snack.

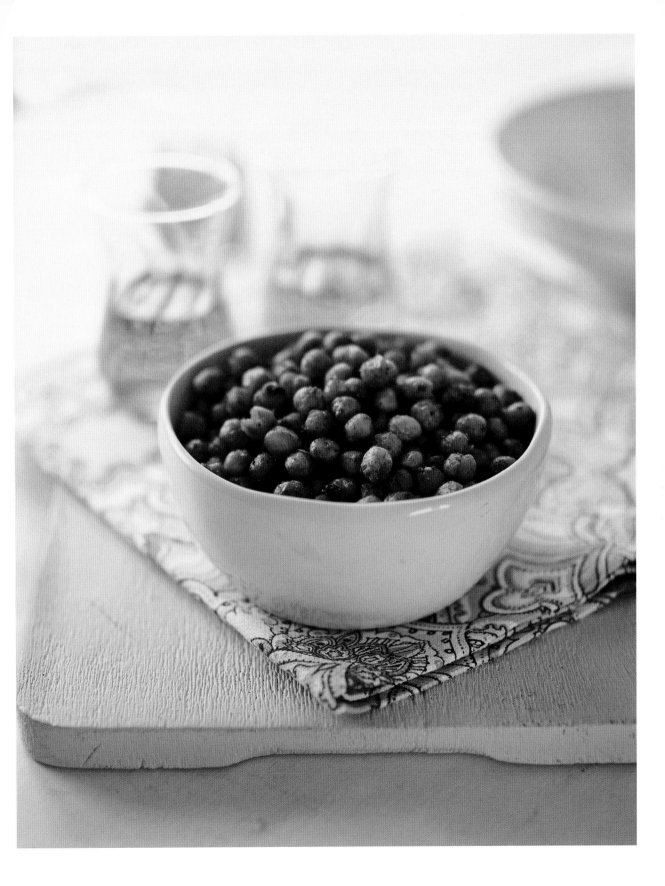

Courgette & Mint Fritters

3 courgettes, coarsely grated

4 spring onions, chopped

4 tablespoons chopped mint

125 g (4 oz) self-raising flour

2 eggs, lightly beaten

125 g (4 oz) ricotta cheese

olive oil, for frying

salt and pepper

lemon-flavoured mayonnaise, to serve

Mix the courgettes, spring onions, mint and flour together in a large bowl, then stir in the eggs. Mix well, season with salt and pepper, then gently fold in the ricotta.

Heat a little oil in a large frying pan. Add 4 separate heaped tablespoonfuls of the batter, flatten slightly and cook for about 3 minutes on each side until golden. Transfer the fritters to a baking sheet and keep warm in a low oven while you repeat with the remaining batter, adding a little more oil to the pan as necessary.

Serve the fritters immediately with a spoonful of lemon-flavoured mayonnaise on the side.

- **FOR FETA & COURGETTE FRITTERS**

Follow the recipe above to make the fritters, using 125 g (4 oz) crumbled feta cheese in place of the ricotta. Cook as above and serve with ready-made fresh tomato salsa instead of the mayonnaise.

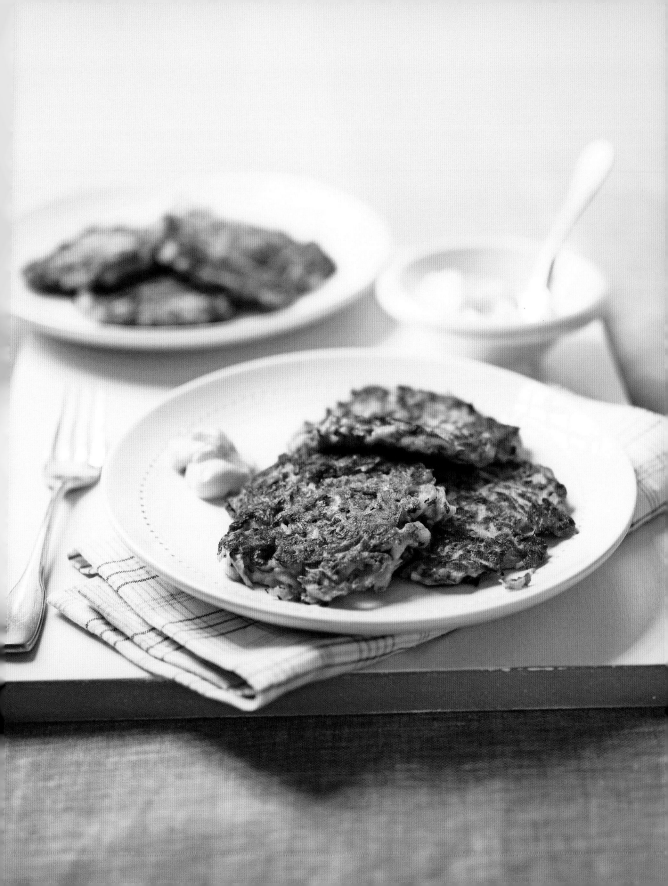

- **SERVES: 4**
- **PREPARATION TIME: 20 MINUTES**
- **COOKING TIME: 4 MINUTES**

Broad Bean Hummus on Goats' Cheese Ciabatta

....

400 g (13 oz) fresh or frozen broad beans

1 garlic clove, crushed

grated rind and juice of 1 lemon

3 tablespoons extra virgin olive oil

125 g (4 oz) goats' cheese

8 slices of ciabatta, toasted

salt and pepper

watercress leaves, to garnish

Cook the broad beans in a saucepan of boiling water for 4 minutes until tender. Drain the beans, then refresh under cold running water and drain again. Slip the beans out of their grey skins, discarding the skins.

Place the beans in a food processor with the garlic and pulse until roughly chopped. Add the lemon rind and juice and then, with the motor running, trickle in the oil through the feed tube. Process until smooth and season to taste with salt and pepper.

Spread a little goats' cheese on each slice of toasted ciabatta, top with the hummus and serve garnished with watercress leaves.

....

- **FOR BROAD BEAN, MINT & MOZZARELLA SALAD**

Cook 200 g (7 oz) broad beans in boiling water and then refresh under cold running water and remove the skins as above. Place the beans in a large bowl and stir in the grated rind and juice of 1 lemon and 2 tablespoons each of chopped mint and olive oil. Cut 2 buffalo mozzarella balls in half and place each half in the centre of a serving plate. Spoon over the broad bean mixture and serve immediately with plenty of freshly ground black pepper and a few mint leaves.

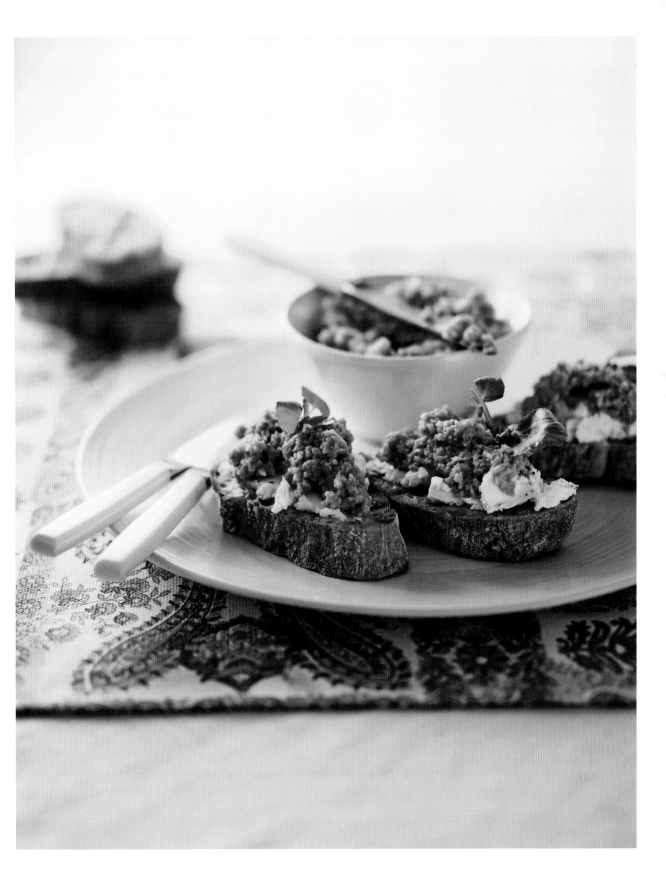

- **SERVES: 6**
- **PREPARATION TIME: 20 MINUTES, PLUS MARINATING AND CHILLING**
- **COOKING TIME: 8–10 MINUTES**

TIP

Fennel contains a phytochemical called anethole; there's some evidence that it has anti-inflammatory and cell-protective properties.

Chicken Tikka Sticks & Fennel Raita

1 onion, finely chopped

½–1 large red or green chilli, deseeded and finely chopped (to taste)

1.5 cm (¾ inch) piece of fresh root ginger, finely chopped

2 garlic cloves, finely chopped

150 g (5 oz) fat-free natural yogurt

3 teaspoons mild curry paste

4 tablespoons chopped coriander

4 chicken breasts, about 150 g (5 oz) each, cubed

Fennel raita

1 small fennel bulb, about 200 g (7 oz)

200 g (7 oz) fat-free natural yogurt

3 tablespoons chopped coriander

salt and pepper

Mix the onion, chilli, ginger and garlic together in a shallow dish. Add the yogurt, curry paste and coriander and mix together.

Add the cubed chicken to the yogurt mixture, mix to coat, cover with clingfilm and chill for at least 2 hours.

Make the raita. Cut the core away from the fennel and finely chop the remainder, including any green tops. Mix the fennel with the yogurt and coriander and season with salt and pepper. Spoon the raita into a serving dish, cover with clingfilm and chill until needed.

Thread the chicken on to 12 skewers and place them on a foil-lined grill rack. Cook under a preheated grill for 8–10 minutes, turning once, or until browned and the chicken is cooked through. Transfer to serving plates and serve with the raita on the side.

- **FOR CHICKEN TIKKA STICKS WITH RED PEPPER & ALMOND CHUTNEY**

Make and cook the chicken skewers as above. Blend 75 g (3 oz) shop-bought roasted peppers in a blender or food processor with a handful of mint leaves, 1 chopped garlic clove and ½ teaspoon chilli powder. Blend until smooth, then add salt to taste and 1½ tablespoons toasted flaked almonds. Pulse a couple of times to roughly crush the almonds and stir in 1 tablespoon chopped coriander. Serve with the skewers.

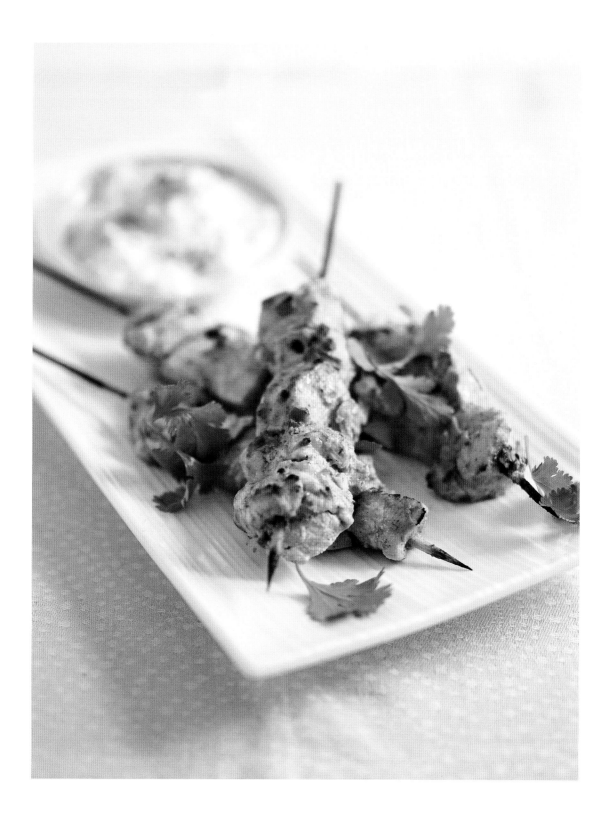

- **SERVES: 2–3**
- **PREPARATION TIME: 8 MINUTES**

Butter Bean & Anchovy Pâté

425 g (14 oz) can butter beans, drained and rinsed

50 g (2 oz) can anchovy fillets in oil, drained

2 spring onions, finely chopped

2 tablespoons lemon juice

1 tablespoon olive oil

4 tablespoons chopped coriander

pepper

4–6 slices of rye bread, toasted, to serve

Place all the ingredients, except the coriander, in a food processor and blend until well mixed but still rough in texture. Alternatively, mash the beans with a fork, finely chop the anchovies and mix the ingredients together by hand.

Stir in the coriander and season well with pepper. Serve with toasted rye bread.

- **FOR BUTTER BEAN & MUSHROOM PÂTÉ**

Cook 250 g (8 oz) sliced mushrooms in 2 tablespoons olive oil with 1 finely chopped garlic clove until the mushrooms are tender and all the liquid has evaporated. Allow to cool, then follow the main recipe, using the mushrooms instead of the anchovies.

- **SERVES: 4**
- **PREPARATION TIME: 10 MINUTES**
- **COOKING TIME: 10 MINUTES**

Chickpea & Sprouted Seed Patties

½ red onion, diced

400 g (13 oz) can chickpeas, rinsed and drained

¼ teaspoon cumin seeds

20 g (¾ oz) sun-dried tomatoes

2 tablespoons sprouted seeds, such as mung or lentil

2 tablespoons olive oil

salt and pepper

To serve

mango chutney

crisp green salad

Place the onion and chickpeas in a blender or food processor and blitz until the chickpeas are broken down. Add all the remaining ingredients except the olive oil, season with salt and pepper and blitz again until the mixture comes together.

Using wet hands, form the mixture into small patties. Cover and chill for 5 minutes.

Heat the oil in a large frying pan, add the patties and cook for 4–5 minutes on each side until golden.

Serve with a little mango chutney and a crisp green salad.

- **SERVES: 4–6**
- **PREPARATION TIME: 10 MINUTES, PLUS COOLING**
- **COOKING TIME: 45–50 MINUTES**

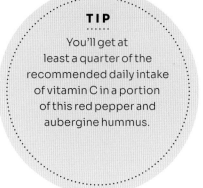

TIP

You'll get at least a quarter of the recommended daily intake of vitamin C in a portion of this red pepper and aubergine hummus.

Pepper & Aubergine Hummus

1 red pepper, cored, deseeded and quartered

3 garlic cloves, unpeeled, lightly crushed

1 aubergine, cut into large chunks

1 tablespoon chilli oil, plus extra to serve

½ tablespoon fennel seeds (optional)

400 g (13 oz) can chickpeas, drained

1 tablespoon tahini

1 teaspoon sesame seeds, lightly toasted

salt and pepper

To serve

4 wholemeal pitta breads

spray oil

1 teaspoon paprika

Put the pepper, garlic and aubergine in a single layer in a large roasting tin. Drizzle with the chilli oil, sprinkle with the fennel seeds, if using, and season with salt and pepper. Place in a preheated oven, 190°C (375°F), Gas Mark 5, for 35–40 minutes or until softened and golden. Remove from the oven but do not turn it off.

Peel the skins from the garlic cloves and put in a food processor or blender with the roasted vegetables, three-quarters of the chickpeas and the tahini. Blend until almost smooth, season to taste and then spoon into a serving bowl. Cover with clingfilm and leave to cool.

Cut the pitta bread into 2.5 cm (1 inch) strips and place in a large bowl. Spray with a little oil and toss with the paprika and a little salt until well coated. Arrange in a single layer on a baking sheet. Toast in the oven for 10–12 minutes or until crisp.

Sprinkle the hummus with the remaining chickpeas and the sesame seeds and drizzle with 1–2 tablespoons chilli oil. Serve with the toasted pitta breads.

- **FOR ROASTED ARTICHOKE & PEPPER HUMMUS**

Replace the aubergine with a drained 400 g (13 oz) can artichoke hearts in water. Roast in the oven with the peppers and garlic, as above, replacing the chilli oil with 1 tablespoon lemon-infused oil. Omit the fennel seeds. Continue as above.

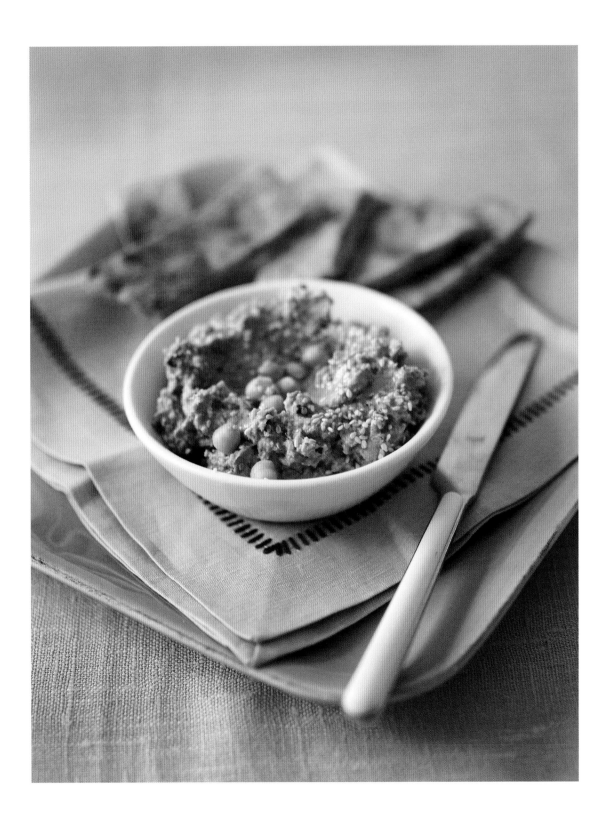

Smoked Trout & Horseradish Pâté

200 g (7 oz) smoked trout

1 teaspoon paprika

2 tablespoons lemon juice

2 tablespoons hot horseradish sauce

100 g (3½ oz) reduced-fat cream cheese

salt and pepper

1 tablespoon snipped chives, to garnish

wholemeal toast or crackers, to serve

Flake the fish, removing any small bones. Place in a food processor with all the remaining ingredients and blend to a coarse pâté, scraping down the sides of the bowl from time to time.

Season to taste, garnish with the chives and serve with wholemeal toast or crackers.

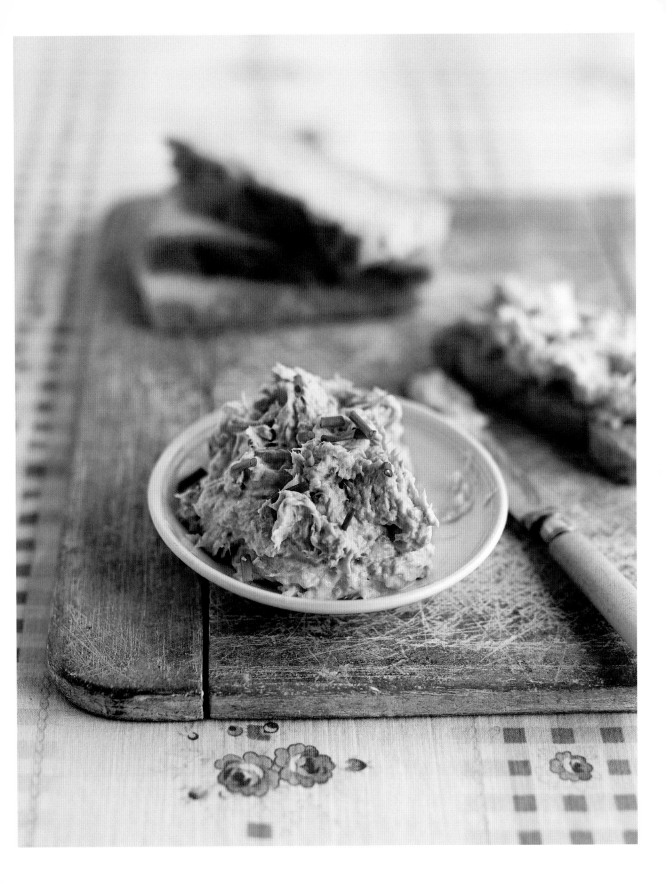

- **SERVES:** 4
- **PREPARATION TIME:** 5 MINUTES
- **COOKING TIME:** 5 MINUTES

Spicy Chilli Chicken Strips

oil, for brushing

350 g (11½ oz) chicken mini breast fillets

lime wedges, to serve

Sauce

2 teaspoons palm sugar or soft brown sugar

1 tablespoon ready-chopped ginger

1 teaspoon lemon grass paste

3 tablespoons sweet chilli sauce

2 tablespoons rice wine vinegar

finely grated rind and juice of 1 lime

4 tablespoons dark soy sauce

Brush a griddle pan with a little oil and heat over a high heat until hot. Meanwhile, cut each chicken fillet in half lengthways. Mix together all the sauce ingredients in a bowl, add the strips of chicken and mix well.

Cook the chicken strips in the hot pan for 3 minutes, brushing with any remaining sauce. Turn over and cook for a further 2 minutes until cooked through. Serve immediately with lime wedges.

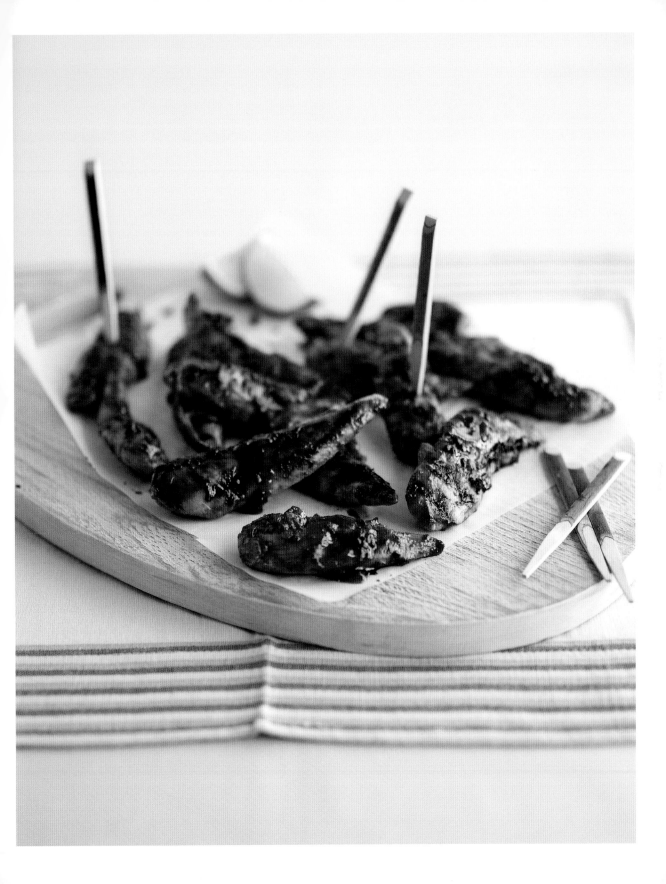

- **SERVES: 4**
- **PREPARATION TIME: 5 MINUTES**
- **COOKING TIME: 8-12 MINUTES**

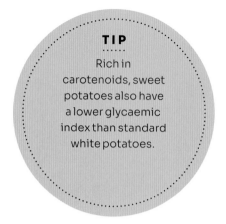

TIP

Rich in carotenoids, sweet potatoes also have a lower glycaemic index than standard white potatoes.

Chilli & Herb Sweet Potato Pancakes

150 g (5 oz) plain flour

3 eggs, lightly beaten

125 ml (4 fl oz) milk

1 tablespoon olive oil

350 g (11½ oz) sweet potatoes, peeled and roughly grated

2 onions, finely sliced

1 red or green chilli, deseeded and finely sliced

4-6 sage leaves, finely chopped

1 tablespoon thyme leaves

sunflower oil, for frying

salt and pepper

sumac, for sprinkling (optional)

Sift the flour into a bowl, make a well in the centre and pour in the eggs. Gradually add the milk, beating continuously to form a smooth batter. Beat in the olive oil. Add the sweet potatoes, onions, chilli, sage and thyme, season well with salt and pepper and mix thoroughly.

Heat a little sunflower oil in a frying pan, swirling it evenly over the base. When hot, pour in 3-4 small ladlefuls of the batter and press each flat. Cook for 2-3 minutes on each side until golden brown, then drain on kitchen paper. Repeat with the remaining batter to make 6-8 pancakes. Serve sprinkled with sea salt or sumac.

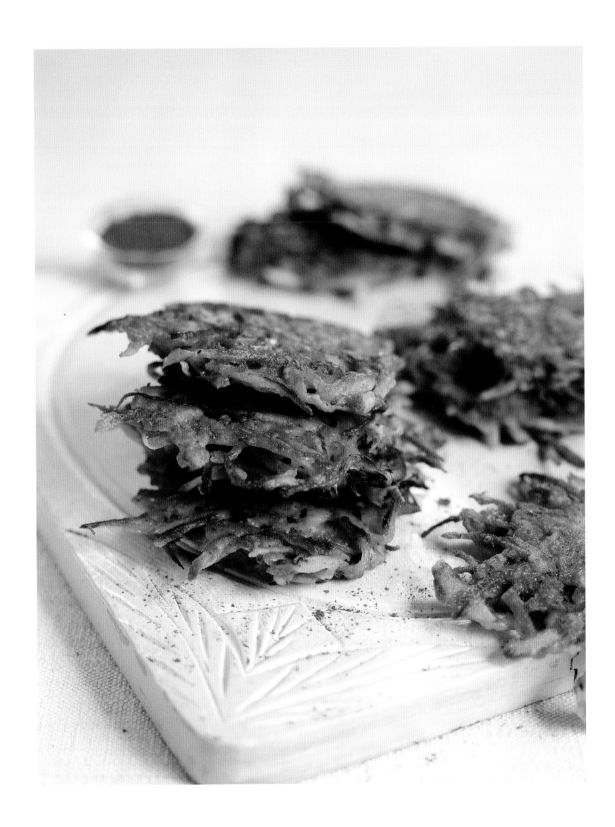

- **SERVES: 4**
- **PREPARATION TIME: 5 MINUTES**
- **COOKING TIME: 2–4 MINUTES**

Greek-style Feta & Mint Dip

150 g (5 oz) feta cheese, crumbled

½ small red onion, thinly sliced

handful of mint leaves, finely chopped

200 ml (7 fl oz) Greek yogurt

pepper

8 wholemeal pitta breads

sliced black olives, to garnish

Mix the cheese with the onion, mint and yogurt, season with black pepper and stir gently to combine. Transfer to a serving bowl and scatter with a few sliced olives.

Cook the pitta breads under a preheated hot grill for 1–2 minutes each side until lightly toasted. Cut into strips and serve with the dip.

- **SERVES: 4**
- **PREPARATION TIME: 10 MINUTES**
- **COOKING TIME: 20–25 MINUTES**

Crisp Parsnip Cakes

750 g (1½ lb) parsnips, peeled and chopped

50 g (2 oz) butter

1 garlic clove, crushed

1 tablespoon chopped thyme

2 tablespoons sunflower oil

salt and pepper

Cook the parsnips in a large saucepan of lightly salted boiling water for 10 minutes until tender.

Meanwhile, melt the butter in a small frying pan, add the garlic and thyme and cook gently, stirring, for 2 minutes.

Drain the parsnips, return to the pan and mash thoroughly. Mash in the buttery garlic mixture and season well with salt and pepper. Leave until cool enough to handle.

Shape the parsnip mixture into 8 patties with lightly floured hands.

Heat 1 tablespoon of the oil in a large frying pan, add 4 of the patties and cook for 3–4 minutes on each side until golden brown. Transfer the patties to a baking sheet and keep warm in a low oven while you repeat with the remaining oil and patties. Serve warm.

- **FOR CURRIED PARSNIP PATTIES**

Cook the parsnips as above. Melt 50 g (2 oz) butter in a frying pan, add 1 crushed garlic clove and 1 tablespoon medium curry powder and cook, stirring, for 2 minutes. Drain the parsnips, return to the pan and mash thoroughly. Beat in the spiced butter mixture with 2 tablespoons chopped coriander. Shape into patties and fry as above.

- **SERVES: 4**
- **PREPARATION TIME: 10 MINUTES**

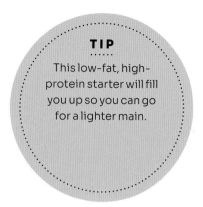

TIP

This low-fat, high-protein starter will fill you up so you can go for a lighter main.

Prawns with Spicy Dip

2 Little Gem lettuces, leaves separated

400 g (13 oz) cooked peeled king prawns

Spicy dip

200 g (7 oz) reduced-fat cream cheese

100 g (3½ oz) natural yogurt

1 garlic clove, crushed

2–3 drops of lemon juice

¼ teaspoon dried chilli flakes

handful of snipped chives

salt and pepper

Make the spicy dip. Mix together the cream cheese, yogurt, garlic, lemon juice, chilli flakes and chives in a serving bowl. Season with salt and pepper to taste.

Arrange the lettuce leaves on 4 small plates and top with the prawns. Serve the dip for everyone to share.

- **FOR SPICY PRAWN SALAD**

Heat 2 tablespoons olive oil in a saucepan, add 1 tablespoon dried chilli flakes and 2 crushed garlic cloves and cook for 2 minutes. Add 500 g (1 lb) raw peeled king prawns and cook for a further 5–6 minutes until the prawns turn pink and are cooked through. Add a splash of white wine and cook until it has evaporated. Remove from the heat. Toss 75 g (3 oz) rocket leaves in 2 tablespoons olive oil and 1 tablespoon balsamic vinegar. Divide between 4 plates and top with 2 peeled, stoned and sliced avocados. Spoon over the prawns and serve sprinkled with 1 tablespoon toasted sesame seeds.

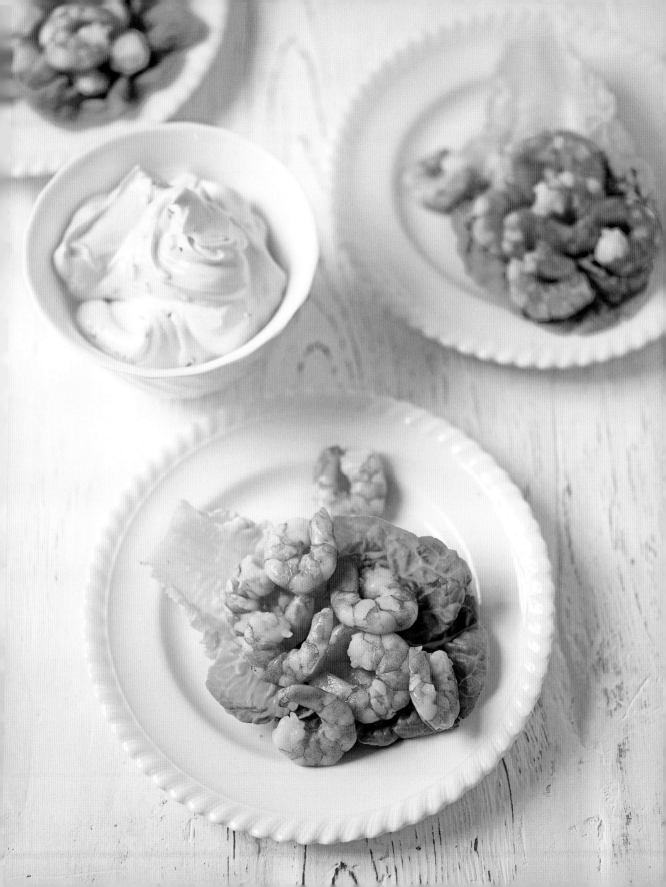

- **SERVES: 4**
- **PREPARATION TIME: 20 MINUTES**
- **COOKING TIME: 12–15 MINUTES**

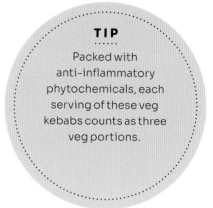

TIP

Packed with anti-inflammatory phytochemicals, each serving of these veg kebabs counts as three veg portions.

Veg Kebabs with Dipping Sauce

3 red onions, cut into wedges

2 courgettes, thickly sliced

2 red peppers, cored, deseeded and chopped

1 yellow pepper, cored, deseeded and chopped

3½ tablespoons olive oil

1 tablespoon balsamic vinegar

2 tablespoons chopped herbs

salt and pepper

Thread the vegetables alternately on to 8 bamboo skewers that have been presoaked in water for 10 minutes to prevent burning. Brush the vegetables with ½ tablespoon of the oil and season well with salt and pepper.

Cook the kebabs under a preheated hot grill or on a barbecue for 12–15 minutes, turning frequently, until tender.

Meanwhile, make the dipping sauce. Mix together the remaining oil, the vinegar and herbs in a small bowl.

Serve the vegetable kebabs with the dipping sauce.

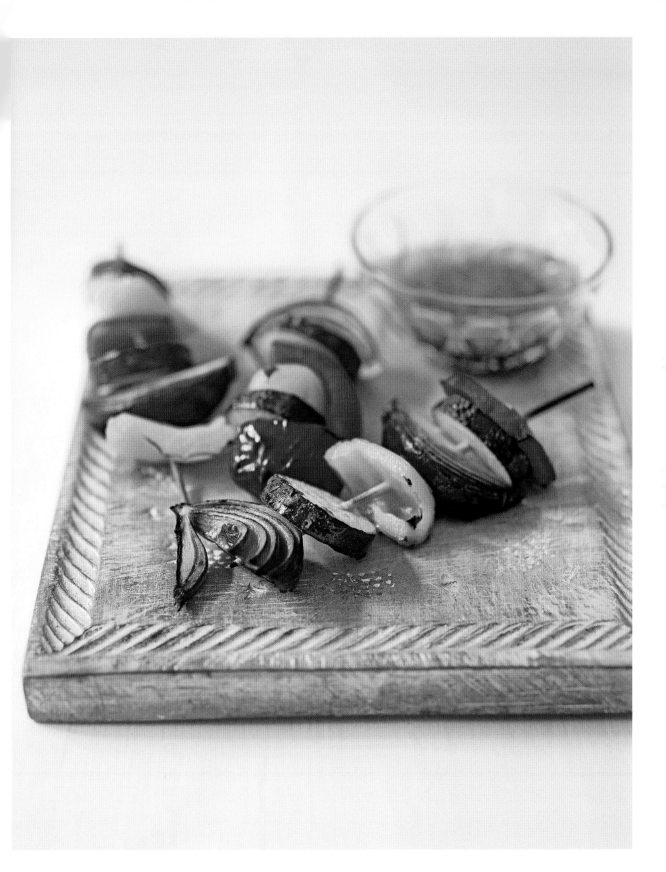

- MAKES: 12–16
- PREPARATION TIME: 15 MINUTES
- COOKING TIME: 10–12 MINUTES

Wholemeal Cheese Straws

....

100 g (3½ oz) wholemeal plain flour, plus extra for dusting

2 teaspoons paprika

150 g (5 oz) mature Cheddar cheese, grated

100 g (3½ oz) chilled unsalted butter, diced

2 teaspoons baking powder

2 egg yolks

Mix together the flour and paprika in a bowl, then stir in the cheese. Add the butter and rub in with the fingertips until the mixture resembles fine breadcrumbs. Stir in the baking powder, then add the egg yolks and mix to a stiff dough.

Turn the dough out on to a floured surface and press or roll out to about 5 mm (¼ inch) thick. Cut into 1 cm (½ inch) wide straws and place on a baking sheet.

Bake in a preheated oven, 220°C (425°F), Gas Mark 7, for 10–12 minutes until golden. Transfer to a wire rack to cool.

TIP

Another delicious opportunity to increase your omega-3 intake, these sesame-coated salmon skewers also provide plenty of antioxidant vitamin E.

Salmon & Sesame Skewers

1 tablespoon soy sauce

2 teaspoons honey

500g (1 lb) salmon fillet, skinned and cut into strips

4 teaspoons sesame oil

juice of 1 lime

1 cucumber

6 spring onions, finely sliced

16 cherry tomatoes, halved

3 tablespoons sesame seeds

Mix together the soy sauce and honey in a shallow bowl. Add the salmon and mix well, then cover and leave to marinate in the refrigerator for 12–15 minutes. Meanwhile, soak 8 wooden skewers in water for 10 minutes.

Mix together the sesame oil and lime juice in a large bowl. Using a vegetable peeler, slice the cucumber into long, thin strips and place in the bowl with the spring onions and cherry tomatoes. Toss the vegetables in the dressing.

Thread the salmon on to the skewers, then roll in the sesame seeds to coat. Cook in a preheated hot griddle pan or under a preheated hot grill for 2–3 minutes on each side or until cooked through.

Serve the salmon skewers with the cucumber salad.

- **MAKES: 12**
- **PREPARATION TIME: 15 MINUTES**
- **COOKING TIME: 10 MINUTES**

Tapenade Bruschetta

....

1 small ciabatta loaf, cut into 12 slices

3 tablespoons olive oil

1 garlic clove, crushed

1 tablespoon chopped flat
leaf parsley

12 marinated sun-dried tomatoes
in oil, drained

Tapenade

150 g (5 oz) pitted black olives

1 garlic clove

small handful of flat leaf parsley

2 tablespoons capers

1 tablespoon lemon juice

2 tablespoons olive oil

salt and pepper

Arrange the ciabatta slices in a single layer on a baking sheet. Mix the oil, garlic and chopped parsley together and brush over the bread slices. Bake in a preheated oven, 200°C (400°F), Gas Mark 6, for 10 minutes until golden and crisp.

Meanwhile, put the olives, garlic, parsley, capers, lemon juice and oil in a food processor and process to a coarse paste. Season with salt and pepper.

Spread the tapenade over the toasts and top each one with a sun-dried tomato.

....

- **FOR ARTICHOKE TAPENADE BRUSCHETTA**

Bake the ciabatta slices as above. Meanwhile, put 75 g (3 oz) pitted green olives, 75 g (3 oz) drained marinated artichokes in oil (reserving 2 tablespoons of the oil), a small handful of flat leaf parsley, 2 tablespoons capers, 1 garlic clove, 1 tablespoon lemon juice and the reserved artichoke oil in a food processor and process to a coarse paste. Season with salt and pepper. Spread the tapenade over the toasts and sprinkle with chopped parsley.

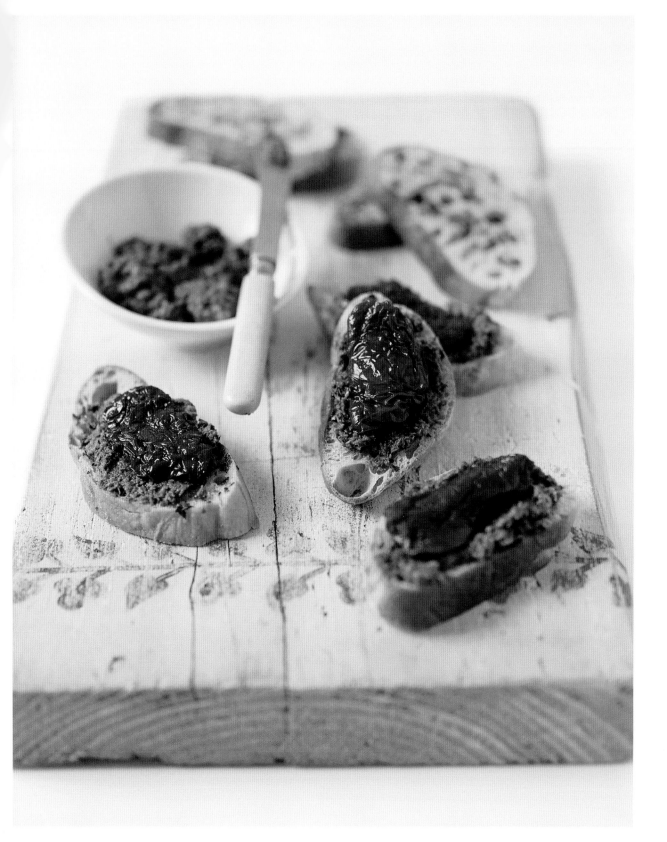

- **SERVES: 4**
- **PREPARATION TIME: 20 MINUTES**
- **COOKING TIME: 35 MINUTES**

Seeded Chips with Red Pepper Dip

450 g (14½ oz) sweet potatoes, peeled and cut into wedges

450 g (14½ oz) white potatoes, peeled and cut into wedges

4 tablespoons olive oil

1 tablespoon poppy seeds

1 tablespoon sesame seeds

1 teaspoon dried chilli flakes

1 large red pepper, cored, deseeded and cut into 4 wedges

2 tomatoes, halved

½ teaspoon smoked paprika

3 tablespoons chopped coriander

salt and pepper

Drizzle the sweet potato and white potato wedges with 3 tablespoons of the olive oil in a large roasting tin and toss well, then scatter over the poppy and sesame seeds and chilli flakes and toss again. Season generously with salt and pepper and roast in the top of a preheated oven, 200°C (400°F), Gas Mark 6, for 35 minutes until golden.

Meanwhile, put the pepper wedges and tomatoes in a smaller roasting tin, then drizzle with the remaining olive oil and toss well. Roast on a lower shelf in the oven for 25 minutes until softened and lightly charred in places.

Transfer the roasted pepper and tomatoes to a food processor, season generously with salt and pepper and add the smoked paprika. Process until almost smooth but with a little texture still remaining. Spoon the mixture into a small serving bowl and place in the centre of a serving platter.

Arrange the roasted potato wedges on the platter, scatter with the chopped coriander and serve.

- **FOR PARSNIP CHIPS WITH HORSERADISH DIP**

Peel 4 large parsnips, cut each into 8 wedges and put in a roasting tin. Toss with 3 tablespoons olive oil and roast in a preheated oven, 200°C (400°F), Gas Mark 6, for 25 minutes until softened and crisp at the edges. Toss with 2 tablespoons maple syrup and 1 tablespoon wholegrain mustard, then arrange on a serving platter and serve with a bowl of horseradish sauce for dipping.

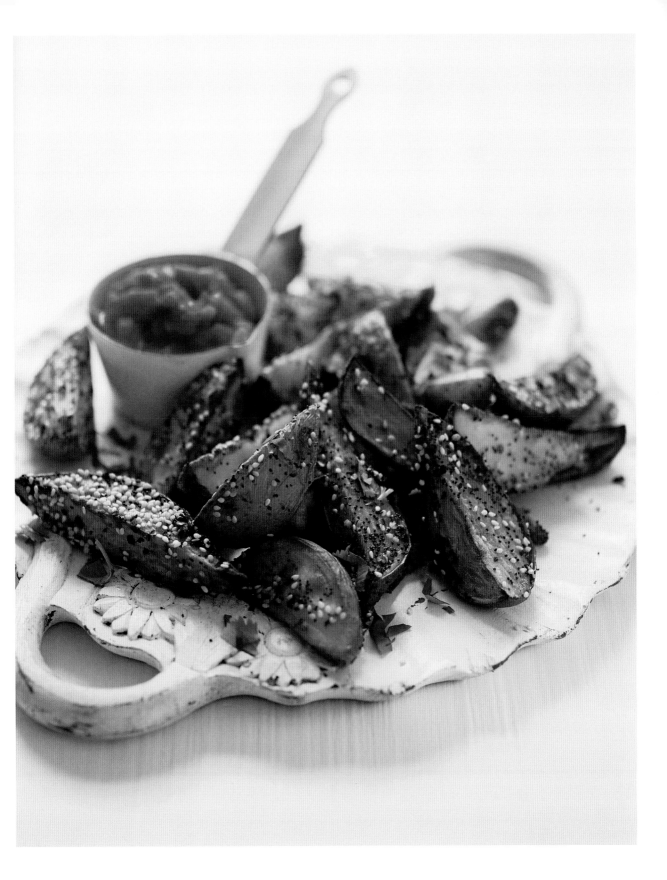

Tasty, Healthy Mains

- **SERVES: 4**
- **PREPARATION TIME: 15 MINUTES**
- **COOKING TIME: 1¾ HOURS**

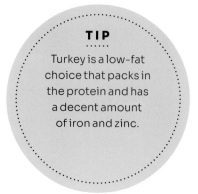

Turkey Chilli

1 tablespoon olive oil

2 red onions, chopped

1 carrot, peeled and diced

1 celery stick, diced

1 red pepper, cored, deseeded and chopped

1 yellow pepper, cored, deseeded and chopped

1 red chilli, deseeded and finely chopped

1 teaspoon smoked paprika

1 teaspoon ground cumin

bunch of coriander, roughly chopped

400 g (13 oz) cooked turkey, roughly chopped or shredded

400 g (13 oz) can butter beans, rinsed and drained

2 x 400 g (13 oz) cans chopped tomatoes

juice of 1 lime

600 g (1¼ lb) cooked rice

Heat the oil in a flameproof casserole dish, add the onions, carrot, celery, peppers and chilli and cook for 5 minutes. Add the paprika, cumin and chopped stalks of the coriander, and cook for a further 5 minutes, stirring occasionally, until the vegetables are softened. Add the turkey, beans and tomatoes, mix well and cover with a lid.

Transfer to a preheated oven, 180°C (350°F), Gas Mark 4, and cook for 1½ hours, checking every 30 minutes and adding a little water if it starts to look dry.

Remove from the oven and stir in the lime juice and chopped coriander leaves. Serve with the cooked rice.

- **FOR TURKEY & RICE NOODLE STIR-FRY**

Cook 300 g (10 oz) rice noodles according to the packet instructions. Heat 1 teaspoon sunflower oil in a wok and fry 400 g (13 oz) cooked turkey, sliced into strips, for 2 minutes. Add 325 g (11 oz) trimmed green beans, 1 sliced red onion and 2 sliced garlic cloves and stir-fry for a further 4–5 minutes. Stir in the juice of 1 lime, 1 teaspoon chilli powder, 1 diced red chilli and 1 tablespoon fish sauce. Add 1 tablespoon chopped mint, 2 tablespoons chopped coriander and the drained rice noodles and toss well before serving.

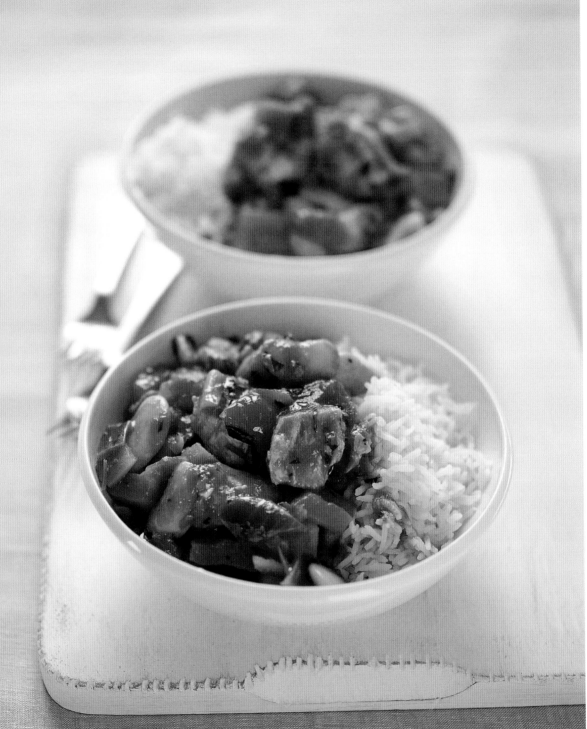

- **SERVES: 4**
- **PREPARATION TIME: 5 MINUTES**
- **COOKING TIME: 10–12 MINUTES**

Penne with Peas & Beans

....

400 g (13 oz) wholewheat penne

1 tablespoon extra virgin rapeseed oil or olive oil

2 spring onions, finely chopped

250 g (8 oz) reduced-fat mascarpone cheese

4 tablespoons lemon juice

250 g (8 oz) frozen peas, thawed

250 g (8 oz) frozen baby broad beans, thawed

small bunch of basil, roughly chopped, a few leaves reserved for garnish

salt and pepper

Cook the penne in a large saucepan of boiling water for 10–12 minutes, or according to the packet instructions, until al dente.

Meanwhile, heat the oil in a large frying pan over a medium-low heat, add the spring onions and fry for 1–2 minutes or until softened. Stir in the mascarpone, lemon juice, peas, broad beans and basil. Season with salt and pepper to taste and stir for 1–2 minutes or until bubbling.

Drain the penne, reserving 3 tablespoons of the cooking water. Stir the pasta and the reserved liquid into the creamy peas and beans. Serve immediately, garnished with extra basil leaves.

....

• FOR BROAD BEAN & PEA RISOTTO

Melt 25 g (1 oz) butter with 1 tablespoon olive oil and cook the spring onions until softened. Add 350 g (11½ oz) risotto rice and stir for 1–2 minutes or until translucent. Add 200 ml (7 fl oz) white wine, then 1 litre (1¾ pints) boiling vegetable stock, a small ladleful at a time and stirring constantly only adding more once the rice has absorbed the previous ladleful. Continue until all the liquid has been absorbed and the rice is just cooked. This should take about 18 minutes. Stir in the peas, beans and basil 2 minutes before the end of the cooking time. Remove from the heat, stir in 125 g (4 oz) mascarpone and serve immediately.

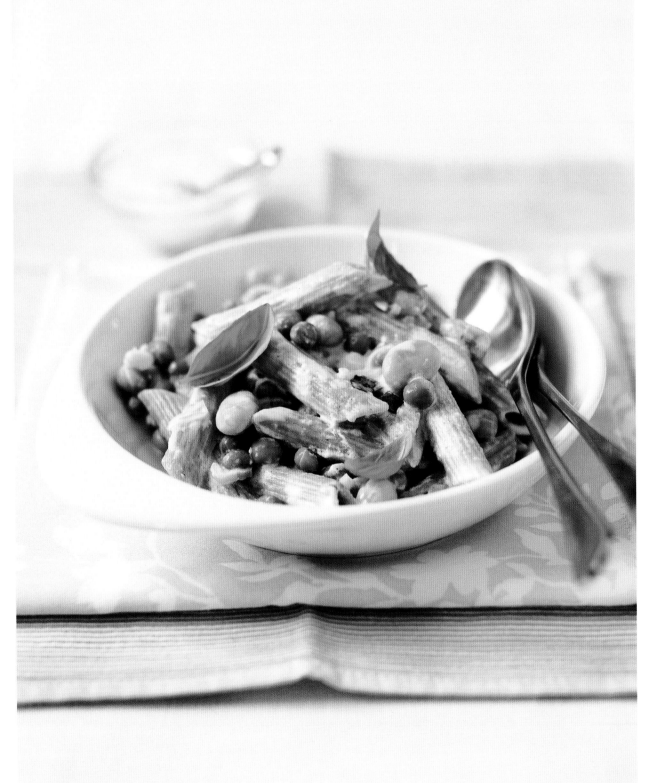

- SERVES: 4
- PREPARATION TIME: 10 MINUTES, PLUS MARINATING
- COOKING TIME: 35–40 MINUTES

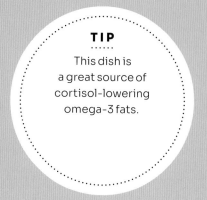

TIP

This dish is a great source of cortisol-lowering omega-3 fats.

Harissa Salmon with Sweet Potato

2 tablespoons natural yogurt

2 teaspoons harissa

2 tablespoons chopped coriander, plus extra to garnish

grated rind and juice of ½ lime

4 pieces of skinless salmon fillet, about 150 g (5 oz) each

vegetable oil, for greasing

lime wedges and flat leaf parsley, to serve

Spicy sweet potato

500 g (1 lb) sweet potato, peeled and cut into chunks

1 tablespoon olive oil

1 teaspoon cumin seeds

½ teaspoon garam masala

salt and pepper

Mix together the yogurt, harissa, coriander and lime rind and juice in a non-metallic bowl. Add the salmon and coat in the mixture. Cover and marinate in the refrigerator for at least 20 minutes.

Toss together the sweet potato chunks, olive oil, cumin seeds and garam masala in a bowl and season well. Put in a roasting tin and place in a preheated oven, 200°C (400°F), Gas Mark 6, for 35–40 minutes until golden.

Heat a lightly greased frying pan or griddle until hot towards the end of the sweet potato roasting time. Add the salmon and cook for 3 minutes on each side until just cooked. Garnish with coriander and serve with the sweet potatoes, lime wedges and flat leaf parsley.

- **FOR SPICED CHICKEN DRUMSTICKS**

Make the yogurt and harissa marinade as above and stir in 1 teaspoon groundnut oil. Pierce the flesh of 8 skinless chicken drumsticks several times, then cover with the marinade. Marinate as above, then place under a hot grill or on a barbecue for 12–15 minutes until cooked through and beginning to char. Serve with a salad.

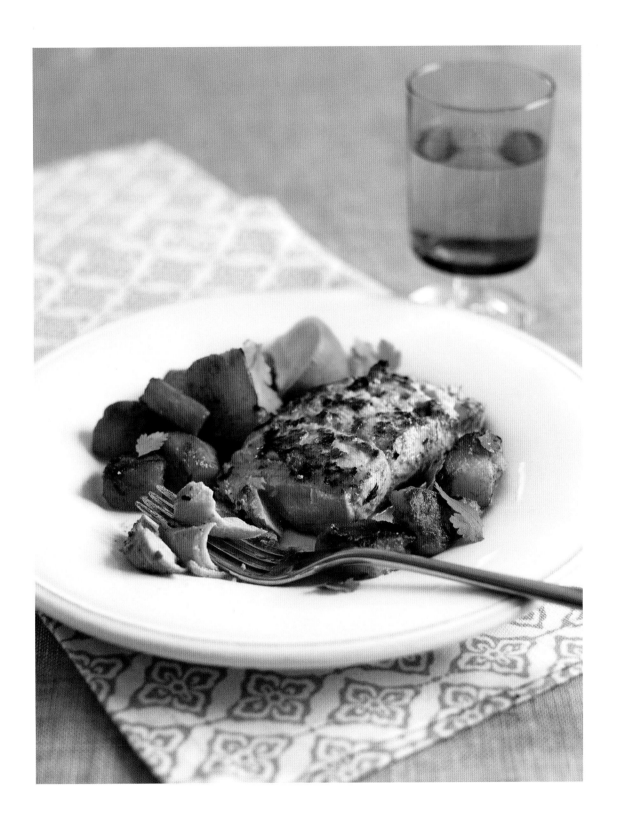

- **SERVES: 4**
- **PREPARATION TIME: 10 MINUTES**
- **COOKING TIME: 25 MINUTES**

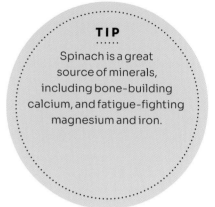

TIP

Spinach is a great source of minerals, including bone-building calcium, and fatigue-fighting magnesium and iron.

Chicken with Spinach & Ricotta

4 boneless, skinless chicken breasts, about 125 g (4 oz) each

125 g (4 oz) ricotta cheese

125 g (4 oz) cooked spinach, squeezed dry

¼ teaspoon grated nutmeg

8 slices of Parma ham

2 tablespoons olive oil, plus extra for drizzling

salt and pepper

To serve

lemon wedges

rocket leaves

Make a long horizontal slit through the thickest part of each chicken breast without cutting right through.

Crumble the ricotta into a bowl. Chop the spinach and mix into the ricotta with the nutmeg. Season with salt and pepper.

Divide the stuffing between the slits in the chicken breasts and wrap each one in 2 pieces of Parma ham, winding it around the chicken to cover the meat totally.

Heat the oil in a shallow ovenproof pan, add the chicken breasts and cook for 4 minutes on each side, or until the ham starts to brown. Transfer to a preheated oven, 200°C (400°F), Gas Mark 6, and cook for 15 minutes until the chicken is cooked through. Serve with lemon wedges and rocket leaves drizzled with olive oil.

- **FOR CHICKEN WITH MOZZARELLA & SUN-DRIED TOMATOES**

Omit the ricotta, spinach and nutmeg, and stuff each chicken breast with a 40 g (1½ oz) slice of mozzarella cheese and a drained piece of sun-dried tomato. Season well with pepper and continue as above.

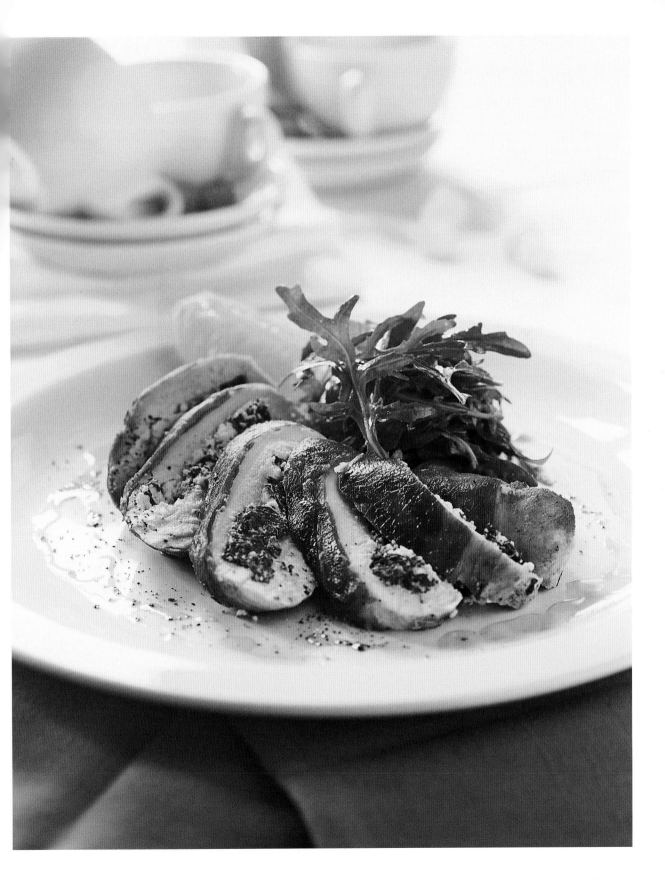

- **SERVES: 4**
- **PREPARATION TIME: 20 MINUTES**
- **COOKING TIME: ABOUT 20 MINUTES**

TIP

Choose fully ripe mangos for the maximum amount of carotenoids (these phytochemicals are what give mangoes their orange colour).

Mango & Coconut Curry

300 g (10 oz) fresh coconut, grated

3–4 fresh green chillies, roughly chopped

1 tablespoon cumin seeds

500 ml (17 fl oz) water

3 firm ripe mangoes, peeled, stoned and cubed

1 teaspoon ground turmeric

1 teaspoon chilli powder

300 ml (½ pint) fat-free natural yogurt, lightly whisked

1 tablespoon groundnut oil

2 teaspoons black mustard seeds

3–4 hot dried red chillies

10–12 curry leaves

Place the coconut, fresh chillies and cumin seeds in a food processor with half the measurement water and blend to a fine paste.

Combine the mangoes with the turmeric, chilli powder and the remaining measurement water in a heavy saucepan. Bring to the boil, add the coconut paste and stir to mix well. Cover and simmer over a medium heat for 10–12 minutes, stirring occasionally, until the mixture becomes fairly thick.

Add the yogurt and heat gently, stirring, until just warmed through. Do not let the mixture come to the boil or it will curdle. Remove from the heat and keep warm.

Heat the oil in a small frying pan over a medium-high heat. Add the mustard seeds and as soon as they begin to pop (after a few seconds), add the dried chillies and curry leaves. Stir-fry for a few seconds until the chillies darken. Stir into the mango curry and serve immediately.

- **SERVES: 2**
- **PREPARATION TIME: 10 MINUTES**
- **COOKING TIME: 15 MINUTES**

TIP

Pasta – even white pasta – has a surprisingly low glycaemic index so this dish won't spike your blood sugar unduly.

Pasta with Fennel & Rocket

1 tablespoon olive oil

1 fennel bulb, trimmed and thinly sliced

1 garlic clove, chopped

100 ml (3½ fl oz) dry white wine

4 tablespoons crème fraîche

grated rind and juice of 1 small lemon

50 g (2 oz) rocket leaves

250 g (8 oz) fresh tagliatelle or pappardelle

salt and pepper

grated Parmesan cheese, to serve

Heat the oil in a frying pan, add the fennel and garlic and cook gently for about 10 minutes until the fennel is soft and golden.

Add the wine to the pan and cook until reduced by half. Stir in the crème fraîche, lemon rind and juice and rocket and cook, stirring, until the rocket has wilted. Season to taste with salt and pepper.

Meanwhile, cook the pasta in a large saucepan of lightly salted boiling water for 3–4 minutes, or according to the packet instructions, until al dente. Drain and return to the pan.

Stir the sauce into the cooked pasta and toss well. Season with freshly ground black pepper and serve immediately with the cheese.

- **FOR PENNE WITH FENNEL, CHILLI & BASIL**

Heat 3 tablespoons olive oil in a frying pan, add 2 crushed garlic cloves and a pinch of dried chilli flakes and cook, stirring, for 1 minute. Add 1 trimmed and thinly sliced fennel bulb and cook gently for about 10 minutes until soft and golden. Meanwhile, cook 250 g (8 oz) fresh penne in a large saucepan of lightly salted boiling water for 3–4 minutes, or according to the packet instructions, until al dente. Drain, reserving 2 tablespoons of the cooking water, and return to the pan. Add the fennel mixture and the reserved cooking water. Stir well, then toss in 1 tablespoon shredded basil leaves. Serve immediately, sprinkled with 2 tablespoons grated Parmesan cheese.

- **SERVES: 4**
- **PREPARATION TIME: 15 MINUTES**
- **COOKING TIME: 40 MINUTES**

TIP

Haddock is a great source of iodine which we need for maintaining a healthy thyroid gland and metabolism.

Mediterranean Roasted Fish

5 tablespoons olive oil

2 shallots, thinly sliced

75 g (3 oz) pancetta, chopped

50 g (2 oz) pine nuts

2 teaspoons chopped rosemary, plus several extra sprigs

1 thick slice of white bread, made into breadcrumbs

50 g (2 oz) can anchovies, drained and chopped

2 red onions, thinly sliced

6 tomatoes, cut into wedges

2 haddock fillets, each about 300 g (10 oz), skinned

salt and pepper

Heat 2 tablespoons of the oil in a large roasting pan and fry the shallots and pancetta, stirring frequently, until beginning to colour. Add the pine nuts and chopped rosemary with a little pepper and fry for a further 2 minutes. Drain to a bowl, add the breadcrumbs and anchovies and mix well.

Add the onions to the pan and fry for 5 minutes until slightly softened. Stir in the tomato wedges and remove from the heat. Push to the edges of the pan to leave a space for the fish in the centre.

Check the fish for any stray bones and place one fillet in the pan. Pack the stuffing mixture on top, pressing it firmly on to the fish with your hands. Lay the second fillet on top, skinned-side down, and season with a little salt and pepper.

Drizzle with the remaining oil and place in a preheated oven, 180°C (350°F), Gas Mark 4, for 30 minutes until the fish is cooked through. Test by piercing a thick area with a knife.

- **FOR ROASTED FISH WITH SPINACH & WALNUT SALAD**

Follow the recipe above to roast the fish. Heat 1 tablespoon clear honey in a small frying pan, add 125 g (4 oz) walnuts and stir-fry over a medium heat for 2–3 minutes until glazed. Meanwhile, blanch 250 g (8 oz) green beans in lightly salted boiling water for 3 minutes and drain. Place in a large bowl with 200 g (7 oz) baby spinach. Whisk the following dressing ingredients together and season with salt and pepper: 4 tablespoons walnut oil, 2 tablespoons olive oil and 1–2 tablespoons sherry vinegar. Pour over the leaves, scatter with the walnuts, and serve with the fish.

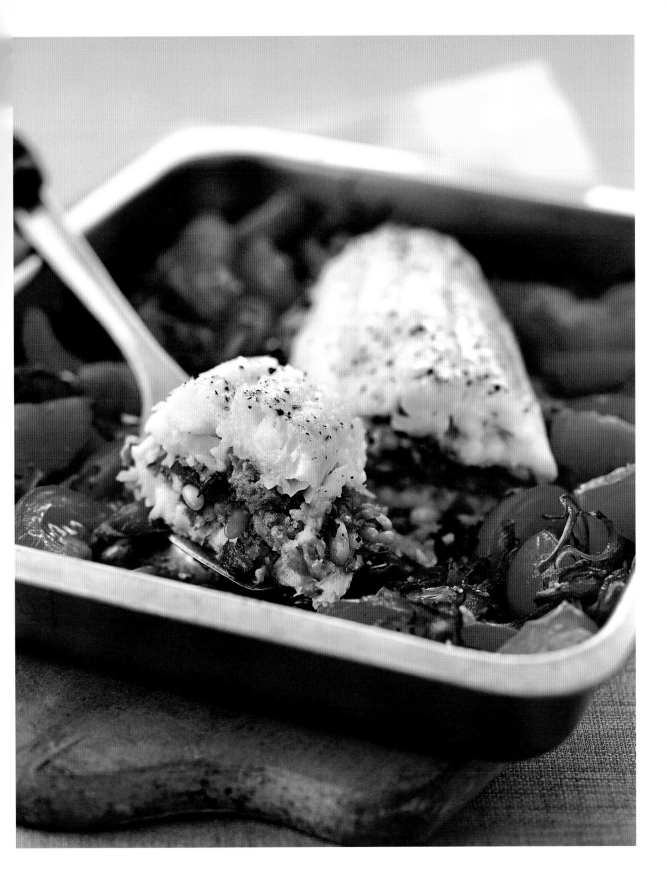

- **SERVES: 4**
- **PREPARATION TIME: 10 MINUTES**
- **COOKING TIME: 45 MINUTES**

Chickpea & Aubergine Tagine

1 tablespoon sunflower oil

1 large onion, sliced

2 garlic cloves, crushed

1 teaspoon ground cumin

1 teaspoon ground cinnamon

1 teaspoon ground turmeric

1 teaspoon ground paprika

2 aubergines, chopped into 3.5 cm (1½ inch) chunks

2 carrots, sliced

125 g (4 oz) ready-to-eat dried dates

400 g (13 oz) can chopped tomatoes

400 g (13 oz) can chickpeas, drained and rinsed

600 ml (1 pint) vegetable stock

4 slices of preserved lemon

2 tablespoons chopped flat leaf parsley

salt and pepper

couscous, to serve

Heat the oil in a large saucepan, add the onion and garlic and cook over a medium heat for 4–5 minutes until softened. Stir in all the spices and cook, stirring, for 1 minute.

Add the aubergines and cook for about 5 minutes until starting to soften. Stir in all the remaining ingredients, except the parsley, and season to taste with salt and pepper.

Bring to the boil, then reduce the heat, cover and simmer for 30 minutes, stirring occasionally.

Stir in the parsley, then serve in warmed deep bowls with couscous.

- **FOR CHICKPEA, APRICOT & ALMOND TAGINE**

Cook the onion and garlic as above, then stir in 2 teaspoons harissa paste and 1 teaspoon ground cinnamon and cook, stirring, for 1 minute. Add the aubergines and cook as above, then add the remaining ingredients, using 125 g (4 oz) ready-to-eat dried apricots in place of the dates. Cook as above, then stir in the parsley, scatter with 50 g (2 oz) toasted blanched almonds and serve with couscous.

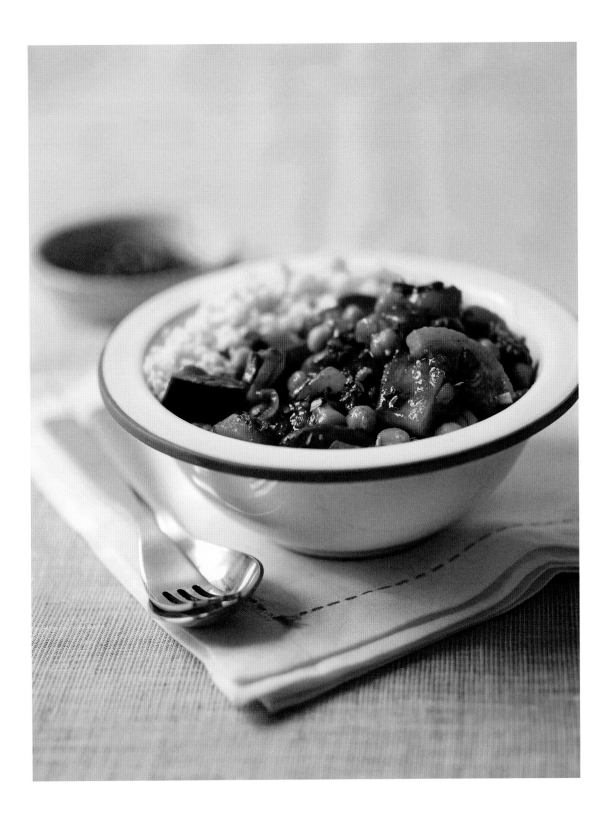

- **SERVES: 4**
- **PREPARATION TIME: 5 MINUTES**
- **COOKING TIME: 7–8 MINUTES**

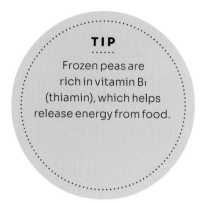

TIP

Frozen peas are rich in vitamin B₁ (thiamin), which helps release energy from food.

Vegetable Broth & Sea Bass

750 ml (1¼ pints) chicken or vegetable stock

1 fennel bulb, cut into 8 wedges, herby tops reserved (optional)

12 fine asparagus spears

150 g (5 oz) frozen peas, thawed

150 g (5 oz) broad beans

2 tablespoons olive oil

4 sea bass fillets, about 200 g (7 oz) each, skin on and pin-boned

small handful of mint leaves, torn

small handful of basil leaves, torn

salt and pepper

Put the stock in a large saucepan and bring to the boil. Add the fennel, reduce the heat and simmer for 3 minutes or until almost tender. Add the asparagus, peas and broad beans and cook for a 1–2 minutes. Season with salt and pepper.

Meanwhile, heat the oil in a frying pan over a medium heat. Season the sea bass with salt and pepper and place, skin side down, in the pan. Cook for 3–4 minutes or until the skin is crispy, then turn the fish over and cook for a further minute.

Ladle the vegetable broth into bowls and sprinkle with a few torn mint and basil leaves. Top the broth with the pan-fried sea bass and reserved herby fennel tops, if using, and serve.

- **FOR THAI-STYLE BROTH WITH PRAWNS**

Peel and devein 500 g (1 lb) raw tiger prawns, reserving the shells and heads. Heat 750 ml (1¼ pints) fish or chicken stock in a saucepan until boiling. Add the prawn shells and heads, 2 roughly chopped lemon grass stalks, a 5 cm (2 inch) piece of fresh root ginger, 1 dried red chilli and 2 kaffir lime leaves. Remove the pan from the heat and leave the stock to infuse for 30 minutes. Strain the stock and return it to a clean saucepan. Add the prawns and poach for 3–4 minutes or until they have turned pink and are cooked through. Add 125 g (4 oz) sugar snap peas 1 minute before the end of the cooking time.

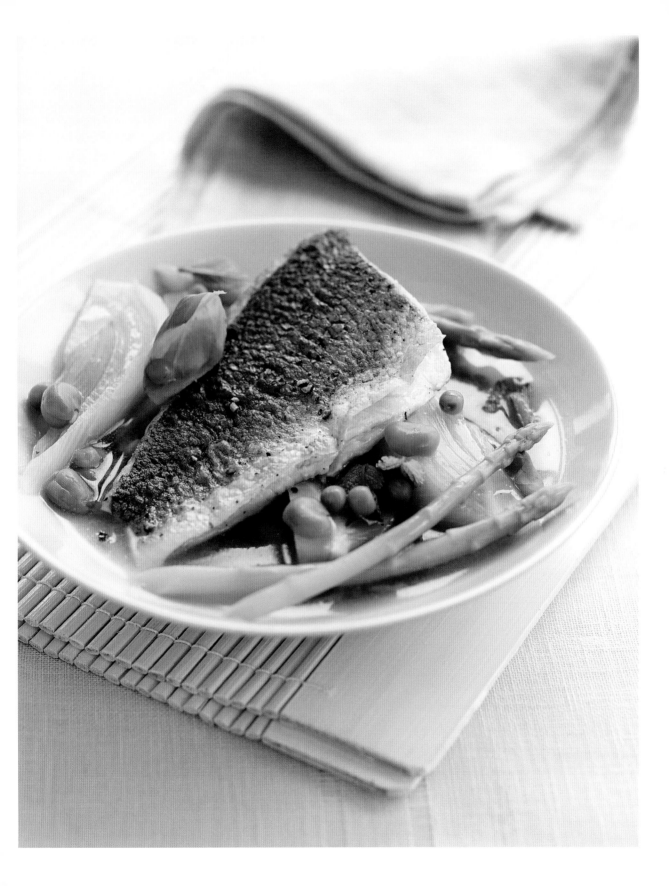

- **SERVES: 4**
- **PREPARATION TIME: 20 MINUTES**
- **COOKING TIME: ABOUT 35 MINUTES**

Chicken & Pickled Walnut Pilaf

400 g (13 oz) boneless, skinless chicken thighs, diced

2 teaspoons Moroccan spice blend (see below for homemade)

4 tablespoons olive oil

50 g (2 oz) pine nuts

1 large onion, chopped

3 garlic cloves, sliced

½ teaspoon ground turmeric

250 g (8 oz) mixed long-grain and wild rice

300 ml (½ pint) chicken stock

3 pieces of stem ginger, finely chopped

3 tablespoons chopped parsley

2 tablespoons chopped mint

50 g (2 oz) pickled walnuts, sliced

salt and pepper

Mix the chicken with the spice blend and a little salt in a bowl.

Heat the oil in a large frying pan over a medium heat, add the pine nuts and fry until beginning to colour. Remove with a slotted spoon and drain on kitchen paper. Add the chicken to the pan and fry gently for 6–8 minutes, or until lightly browned, stirring occasionally.

Stir in the onion and fry for 5 minutes. Add the garlic and turmeric and fry for a further 1 minute. Add the rice and stock and bring to the boil, then reduce the heat to low and simmer very gently for about 15 minutes or until the chicken is cooked through, the rice is tender and the stock absorbed. Add a little water if the liquid has been absorbed before the rice is cooked through.

Stir in the ginger, parsley, mint, walnuts and pine nuts. Season with salt and pepper to taste and heat through gently for 2 minutes before serving.

- **FOR A HOMEMADE SPICE BLEND**

Mix together ½ teaspoon each of crushed fennel, cumin, coriander and mustard seeds with ¼ teaspoon each of ground cloves and ground cinnamon.

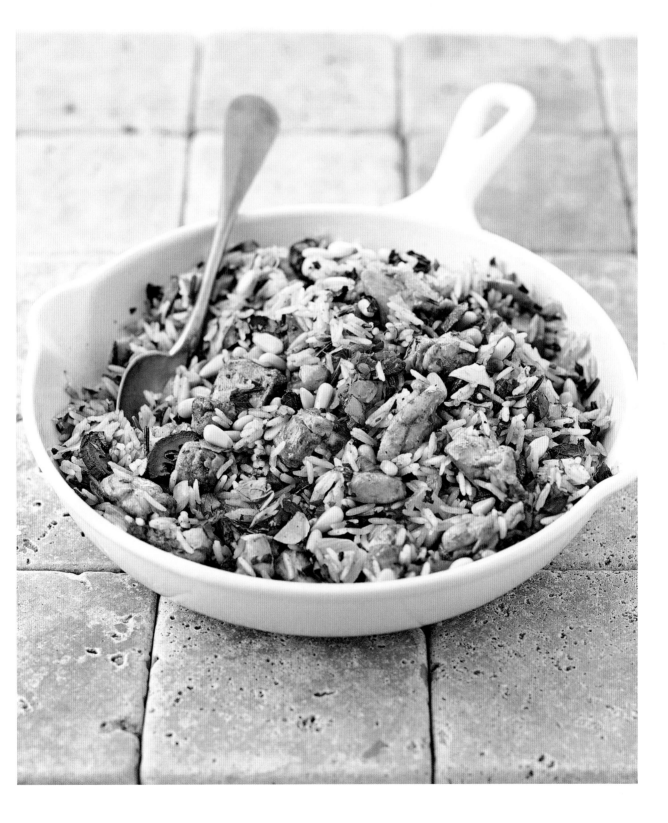

- **SERVES: 4**
- **PREPARATION TIME: 15 MINUTES**
- **COOKING TIME: ABOUT 1 HOUR 10 MINUTES**

TIP

A much-underrated grain, barley is a slow-releasing carb that can help lower cholesterol. It also provides iron to protect against anemia.

Chicken & Barley Risotto

2 tablespoons olive oil

6 boneless, skinless chicken thighs, diced

1 onion, roughly chopped

2 garlic cloves, finely chopped

200 g (7 oz) chestnut mushrooms, sliced

250 g (8 oz) pearl barley

200 ml (7 fl oz) red wine

1.2 litres (2 pints) chicken stock

salt and pepper

parsley leaves, to garnish

To serve

Parmesan cheese shavings

garlic bread (optional)

green salad (optional)

Heat the oil in a large frying pan over a medium-high heat, add the chicken and onion and fry for 5 minutes, stirring until lightly browned.

Stir in the garlic and mushrooms and fry for 2 minutes, then mix in the pearl barley. Add the red wine and half the stock and season with plenty of salt and pepper, then bring to the boil, stirring continuously. Reduce the heat, cover and simmer for 1 hour, topping up with extra stock as needed, until the chicken is cooked through and the barley is soft.

Spoon into shallow bowls, garnish with the parsley and sprinkle with Parmesan. Serve with garlic bread and green salad, if liked.

- **FOR CHICKEN & RED RICE RISOTTO**

Fry the chicken and 1 chopped red onion as above. Add the garlic and 200 g (7 oz) skinned and diced tomatoes, omitting the mushrooms and pearl barley. Stir in 250 g (8 oz) red Camargue rice, cook for 1 minute, then add the red wine. Gradually add the hot stock a small ladleful at a time and stirring constantly, only adding more once the rice has absorbed the previous ladleful. Continue until all the liquid has been absorbed and the chicken and rice are tender. This should take about 25 minutes. Crumble 125 g (4 oz) St Agur or Roquefort cheese on top.

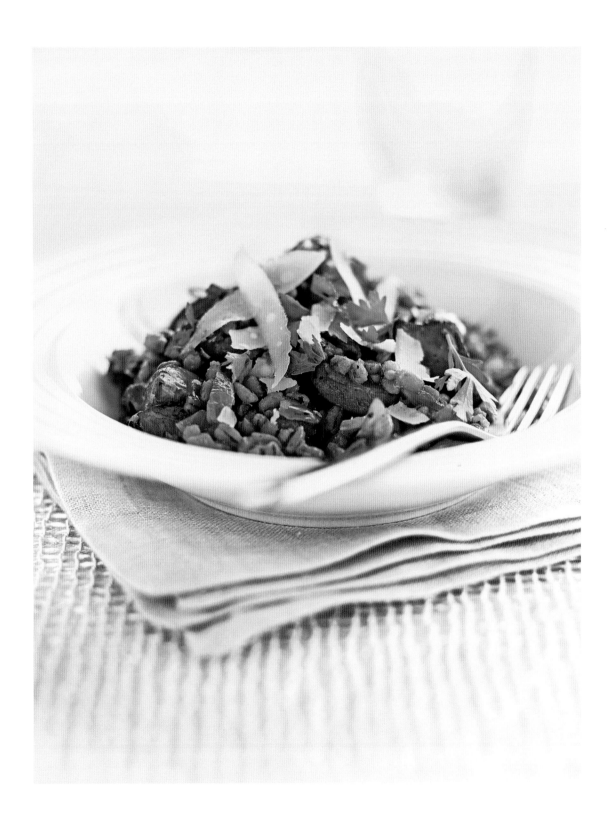

- **SERVES: 4**
- **PREPARATION TIME: 10 MINUTES**
- **COOKING TIME: 15–20 MINUTES**

Mackerel Curry

1 green chilli, deseeded and chopped

1 teaspoon ground coriander

½ teaspoon turmeric

4 garlic cloves, peeled

2.5 cm (1 inch) piece of fresh root ginger, peeled and sliced

1 teaspoon sunflower oil

1 tablespoon coconut oil

1 teaspoon cumin seeds

1 large onion, sliced

150 ml (¼ pint) coconut milk

250 ml (8 fl oz) water

450 g (14½ oz) mackerel fillets, cut into 5 cm (2 inch) pieces

small handful of coriander leaves, roughly torn

salt and pepper

Place the chilli, ground coriander, turmeric, garlic, ginger and sunflower oil in a blender or food processor and blend together to make a smooth paste.

Heat the coconut oil in a wok or frying pan over a medium heat, add the spice paste and the cumin seeds and cook for 2–3 minutes.

Add the onion to the pan and cook for 1–2 minutes, then pour in the coconut milk and measured water. Bring to the boil, then reduce the heat and simmer for 5 minutes. Season with salt and pepper.

Add the mackerel pieces to the pan and cook for 6–8 minutes until the fish is cooked through, then stir in the coriander leaves.

- **FOR MACKEREL, BEETROOT & HORSERADISH SALAD**

Cut 425 g (14 oz) raw beetroot into 4–6 wedges each, place in a roasting tin with 2 tablespoons olive oil, 2 teaspoons cumin seeds, 2 tablespoons thyme and 2 teaspoons clear honey and mix to coat. Roast in a preheated oven, 200°C (400°F), Gas Mark 6, for 25 minutes until tender. Meanwhile, whisk together 2 tablespoons creamed horseradish, 4 tablespoons lemon juice and 150 ml (¼ pint) low-fat natural yogurt in a small bowl. Heat 375 g (12 oz) smoked mackerel fillets according to the packet instructions, then flake into large flakes. Place a few small handfuls of baby spinach leaves on to 4 plates and scatter over the mackerel and beetroot. Sprinkle with the horseradish dressing and serve.

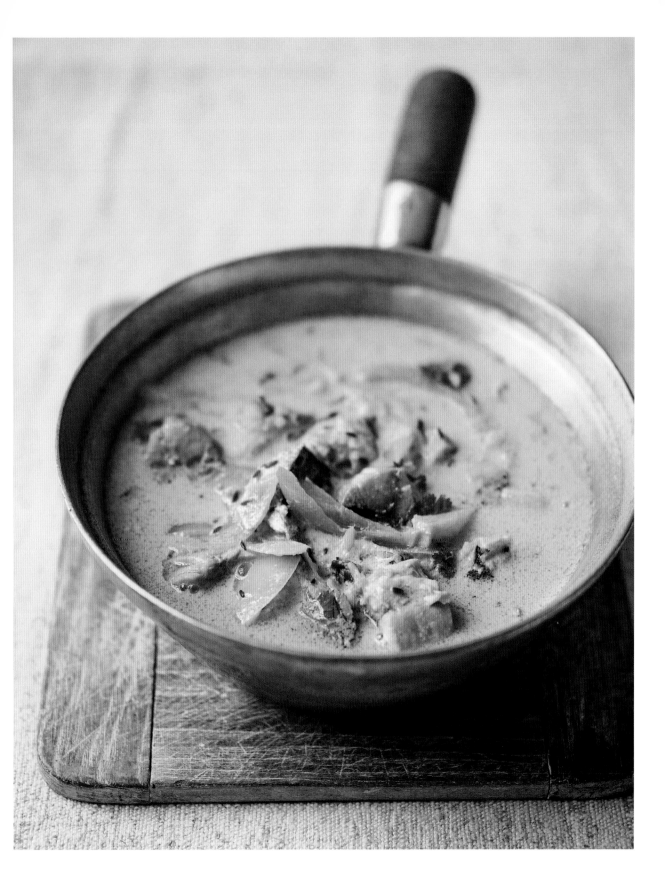

- **SERVES: 4**
- **PREPARATION TIME: 20 MINUTES**
- **COOKING TIME: 55 MINUTES**

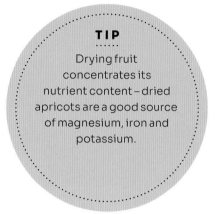

TIP

Drying fruit concentrates its nutrient content – dried apricots are a good source of magnesium, iron and potassium.

Speedy Spiced Chicken Tagine

1 tablespoon olive oil

8 skinless chicken thighs

1 onion, sliced

2 garlic cloves, finely chopped

500 g (1 lb) plum tomatoes, cut into chunks

1 teaspoon ground turmeric

1 cinnamon stick, halved

2.5 cm (1 inch) piece of fresh root ginger, grated

2 teaspoons runny honey

100 g (3½ oz) ready-to-eat dried apricots, quartered

200 g (7 oz) couscous

450 ml (¾ pint) boiling water

grated rind and juice of 1 lemon

small bunch of coriander, roughly chopped

salt and pepper

Heat the oil in a large frying pan, add the chicken and fry until browned on both sides. Lift out and transfer to a tagine or casserole dish. Add the onion to the pan and fry until golden.

Stir in the garlic, tomatoes, spices and honey. Add the apricots and a little salt and pepper and heat through. Spoon over the chicken, cover the dish and bake in a preheated oven, 180°C (350°C), Gas Mark 4, for 45 minutes or until the chicken is cooked through.

When the chicken is almost ready, soak the couscous in the boiling water for 5 minutes. Stir in the lemon rind and juice, coriander and seasoning. Spoon onto plates and top with the chicken and tomatoes, discarding the cinnamon stick just before eating.

- **FOR CHICKEN & VEGETABLE TAGINE**

Use just 4 chicken thighs and add 1 diced carrot, 1 cored, deseeded and diced red pepper and 150 g (5 oz) frozen broad beans. Replace the cinnamon with 2 teaspoons harissa paste and add 150 ml (¼ pint) chicken stock. Cook as above, adding 100 g (3½ oz) thickly sliced okra or green beans for the last 15 minutes of cooking. Sprinkle with chopped coriander or mint and serve with rice.

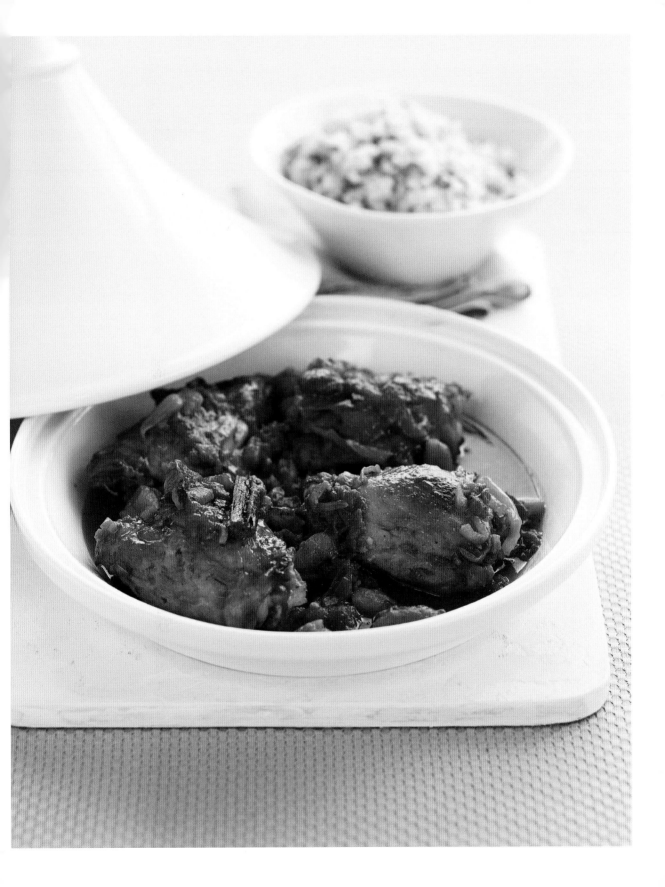

- **SERVES: 4**
- **PREPARATION TIME: 25 MINUTES**
- **COOKING TIME: 1 HOUR 5 MINUTES**

Turkish-style Stuffed Butternut Squash

2 butternut squash, halved and deseeded

4 tablespoons olive oil

salt and pepper

Filling

3 tablespoons olive oil

1 large onion, finely chopped

1 garlic clove, thinly sliced

1 teaspoon ground cumin

450 g (14½ oz) tomatoes, roughly chopped

4 tablespoons chopped flat leaf parsley

1 tablespoon chopped oregano

2 tablespoons sun-dried tomato paste

1 teaspoon cumin seeds

salt and pepper

rocket salad, to serve (optional)

Sit the squash halves, cut-side up, in a large roasting tin, brush each with 1 tablespoon oil and season with salt and pepper. Roast in a preheated oven, 220°C (425°F), Gas Mark 7, for 45 minutes until lightly charred on top.

Meanwhile, heat the oil for the filling in a large, heavy-based frying pan, add the onion, garlic and cumin and cook over a medium-high heat, stirring occasionally, for 4–5 minutes until beginning to soften. Add the tomatoes, parsley, oregano and sun-dried tomato paste and cook, stirring occasionally, for a further 5 minutes. Season well with salt and pepper.

Divide the filling between the cavities of the squash halves and scatter with the cumin seeds. Reduce the oven temperature to 180°C (350°F), Gas Mark 4, and roast the stuffed squash for 20 minutes, or until the filling is soft and golden in places. Serve with a rocket salad if liked.

- **FOR TURKISH-STYLE STUFFED PEPPERS WITH RAISINS**

Heat 4 tablespoons olive oil in a large frying pan, add 2 roughly chopped onions, 2 thinly sliced garlic cloves and 2 teaspoons ground cumin and cook over a medium-high heat, stirring occasionally, for about 8 minutes until the onions are soft. Stir in 750 g (1½ lb) roughly chopped tomatoes, 5 tablespoons raisins, 4 tablespoons chopped flat leaf parsley and 2 tablespoons sun-dried tomato paste, then cover and cook for a further 5 minutes. Season with salt and pepper. Fill 4 cored, deseeded and halved peppers with the mixture in a roasting tin, cover with foil and bake in a preheated oven, 180°C (350°F), Gas Mark 4, for 20 minutes. Remove the foil and cook for a further 10 minutes.

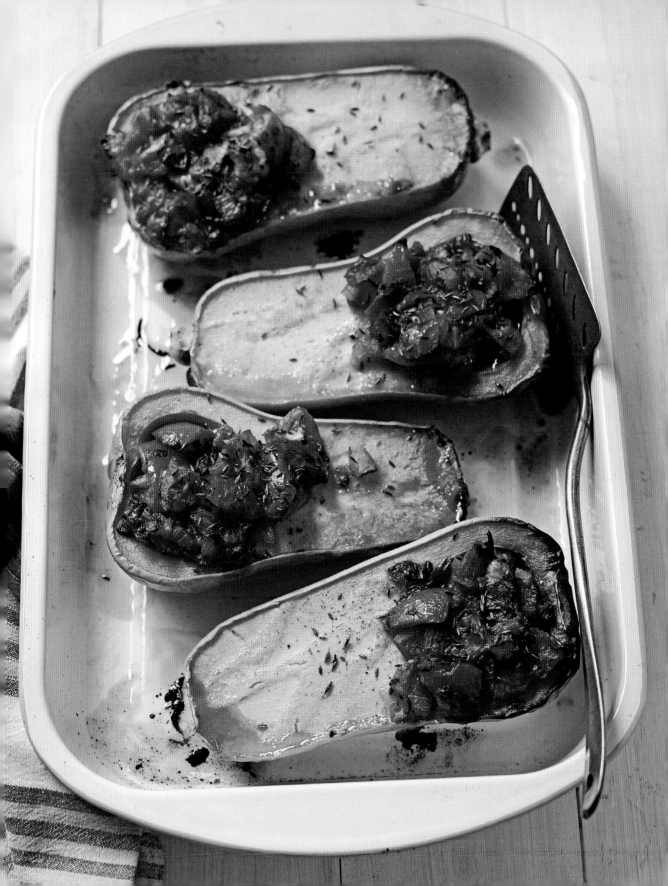

- **SERVES: 4**
- **PREPARATION TIME: 20 MINUTES, PLUS PROVING**
- **COOKING TIME: 45 MINUTES**

Artichoke & Asparagus Pizzas

TIP

A wholegrain base and plenty of vegetable topping make these pizzas nutritionally far superior to the fast-food kind!

400 g (13 oz) wholemeal flour

5 g (¼ oz) fast-action dried yeast

2 teaspoons sugar, plus a pinch

1½ teaspoons salt

2 tablespoons olive oil

225 ml (7½ fl oz) hand-hot water

2 garlic cloves, finely chopped

300 g (10 oz) basil and onion passata

1½ teaspoons dried oregano

400 g (13 oz) can artichokes in water, drained and thickly sliced

200 g (7 oz) asparagus tips

250 g (8 oz) ricotta cheese

100 g (3½ oz) finely grated reduced-fat extra mature Cheddar cheese (optional)

handful of rocket leaves

chilli oil, for drizzling (optional)

salt and pepper

Put the flour, yeast, 2 teaspoons sugar and the salt in a bowl. Pour in 1 tablespoon of the oil and measurement water and mix to a dough. Turn the dough out onto a lightly floured surface and knead for 4–5 minutes until smooth and elastic. Place in a lightly oiled bowl, cover with oiled clingfilm and leave in a warm place for 1½ hours or until doubled in size.

Meanwhile, heat the remaining oil in a saucepan over a low heat, add the garlic and cook for 1 minute. Stir in the passata, ½ teaspoon of the oregano and a pinch of sugar and season with salt and pepper to taste. Simmer for 30 minutes or until thick. Heat a griddle pan, add the artichokes and cook for 3–4 minutes, turning once, or until slightly charred. Repeat with the asparagus.

Divide the dough into 4 and roll out each piece on a floured surface until about 20 cm (8 inches) in diameter. Place the bases on lightly greased baking sheets, cover and leave to rise for a further 30–45 minutes. Thinly spread the sauce over the bases and arrange the griddled vegetables on top. Add teaspoons of ricotta and the Cheddar, if using. Scatter over the remaining oregano.

Place in a preheated oven, 200°C (400°F), Gas Mark 6, for 12–15 minutes or until bubbling and the bases are crisp. Serve topped with the rocket and drizzled with a little chilli oil, if liked.

- **FOR QUICK PITTA PIZZAS**

Spread a little basil and garlic passata over 4 wholemeal pitta breads. Top with 200 g (7 oz) char-grilled vegetables and the ricotta, Cheddar and oregano, as above. Place under a preheated grill for 4–5 minutes or until golden and bubbling.

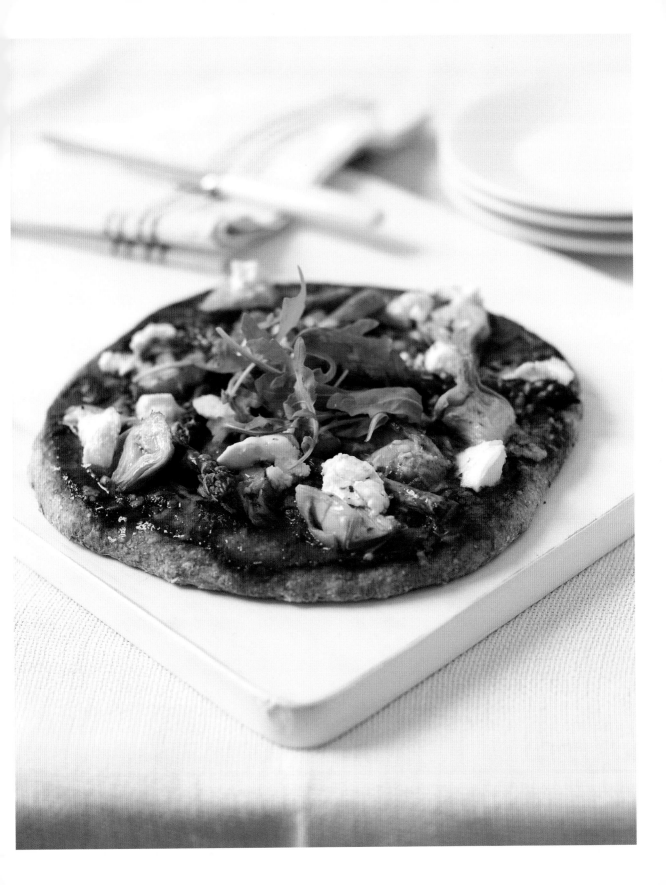

- **SERVES: 4**
- **PREPARATION TIME: 15 MINUTES**
- **COOKING TIME: 55 MINUTES**

Moroccan-style Fish Tagine

750 g (1½ lb) firm white fish fillets, such as cod, sea bass or monkfish, pin-boned, skinned and cut into 5 cm (2 inch) chunks

½ teaspoon cumin seeds

½ teaspoon coriander seeds

6 cardamom pods

4 tablespoons olive oil

2 small onions, thinly sliced

2 garlic cloves, crushed

¼ teaspoon ground turmeric

1 cinnamon stick

40 g (1½ oz) sultanas

25 g (1 oz) pine nuts, lightly toasted

150 ml (¼ pint) fish stock

finely grated rind of 1 lemon, plus 1 tablespoon juice

salt and pepper

Season the fish with salt and pepper.

Using a pestle and mortar, crush the cumin and coriander seeds and cardamom pods. Discard the cardamom pods, leaving the cardamom seeds in the mortar.

Heat the oil in a large, shallow frying pan and fry the onions gently for 6–8 minutes until golden. Add the garlic, crushed spices, turmeric and cinnamon and fry gently, stirring, for 2 minutes. Add the fish pieces, turning them until they are coated in the oil. Transfer the fish and onions to an ovenproof casserole dish and scatter with the sultanas and pine nuts.

Add the stock and lemon rind and juice to the frying pan and bring the mixture to the boil. Pour the mixture around the fish, then cover and bake in a preheated oven, 160°C (325°F), Gas Mark 3, for 40 minutes.

- **FOR FISH TAGINE WITH POMEGRANATE & CORIANDER COUSCOUS**

Make the fish tagine as above. Bring 400 ml (14 fl oz) vegetable stock to the boil. Pour it over 300 g (10 oz) couscous in a heatproof bowl, cover and leave to steam for 5 minutes, then stir in the seeds of 1 pomegranate and 2 tablespoons roughly chopped coriander leaves. Finally, mix in 2 tablespoons olive oil and the juice of ½ lemon and season with salt and pepper.

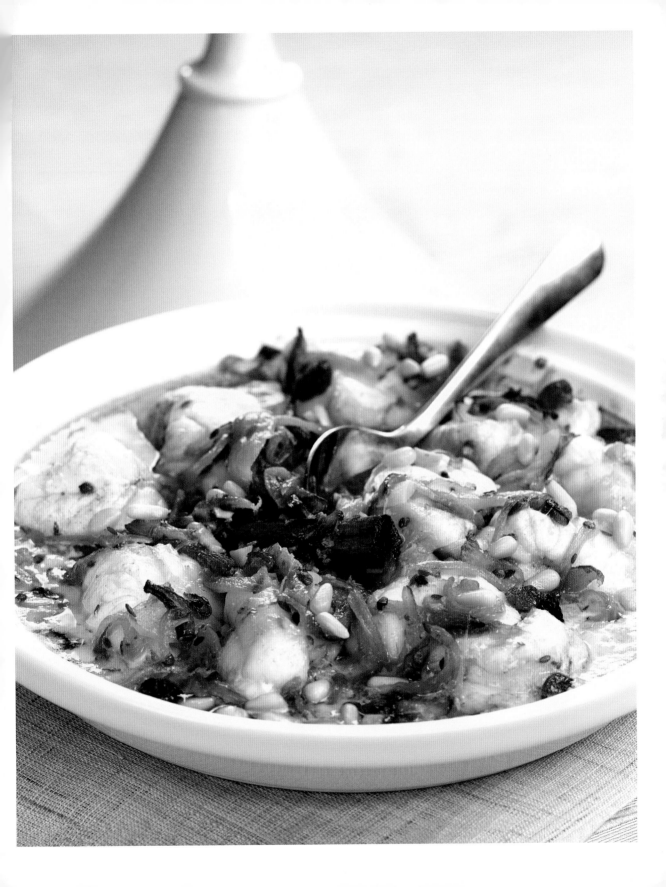

- **SERVES: 4**
- **PREPARATION TIME: 15 MINUTES**
- **COOKING TIME: 8–11 MINUTES**

TIP

This dish is packed with good fats, protein and fibre to help keep your heart, muscles and digestive system healthy. Add a carb-packed side such as the Baked Carrot & Potato Tagine on page 186 for a more substantial meal.

Grilled Salmon with Kale Salad

1 tablespoon sunflower seeds

200 g (7 oz) kale, shredded

4 salmon fillets, about 150 g (5 oz) each

¼ small red cabbage, shredded

1 carrot, peeled and cut into matchsticks

1 avocado, peeled, stoned and sliced

100 g (3½ oz) cherry tomatoes, halved

2 tablespoons extra virgin olive oil

juice of ½ lime

½ teaspoon Dijon mustard

½ teaspoon maple syrup

2 tablespoons chopped chives

pepper

Heat a nonstick frying pan over a medium-low heat and dry-fry the sunflower seeds for 2–3 minutes, stirring frequently, until slightly golden and toasted. Set aside.

Place the kale in a colander, then pour over boiling water to slightly wilt the kale. Refresh under cold running water and drain.

Cook the salmon fillets under a preheated hot grill for 3–4 minutes on each side, or until cooked through.

Meanwhile, toss the kale together with the cabbage, carrot, avocado and tomatoes in a serving bowl. Whisk together the remaining ingredients and pour over the salad.

Scatter the toasted seeds over the salad. Serve the salad with the salmon, sprinkled with a little pepper.

- **FOR GARLIC KALE WITH PAN-FRIED TUNA**

Heat 1 tablespoon sunflower oil in a wok and stir-fry 2 sliced garlic cloves for a few seconds, then add 200 g (7 oz) shredded kale. Toss around in the garlicky oil, then pour over 100 ml (3½ fl oz) boiling water and cook for 5–6 minutes until the kale has wilted. Meanwhile, heat 1 tablespoon olive oil in a separate frying pan and cook 4 x 150 g (5 oz) tuna steaks for 3–4 minutes on each side (depending on how rare you like your tuna). Stir 1 tablespoon soy sauce and 1 tablespoon oyster sauce into the kale and heat through. Serve topped with the tuna.

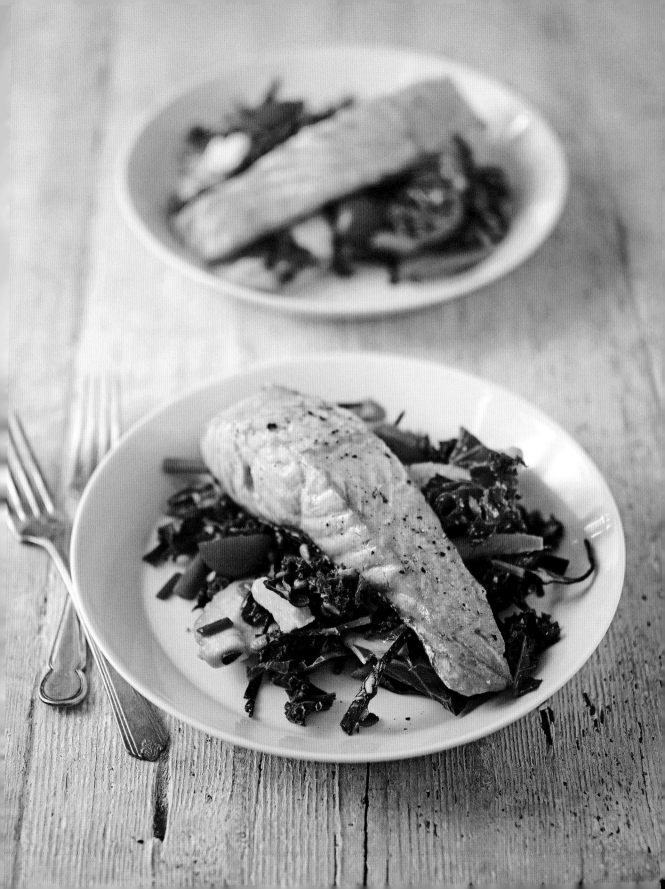

Light Bites & Sides

- **SERVES: 4**
- **PREPARATION TIME: 5 MINUTES**
- **COOKING TIME: 5 MINUTES**

Moroccan-style Vegetable Couscous

....

1 tablespoon harissa paste, plus extra to serve

finely grated rind and juice of 1 lemon

200 g (7 oz) couscous

300 ml (½ pint) boiling water

1 tablespoon olive oil

500 g (1 lb) frozen grilled Mediterranean vegetables, such as aubergine, courgette, peppers and onions

2 preserved lemons, rinsed

400 g (13 oz) can chickpeas, drained and rinsed

small bunch of coriander, roughly chopped

salt and pepper

natural yogurt, to serve

Put the harissa and lemon rind and juice in a large heatproof bowl and add the couscous and boiling water. Stir, cover and leave to stand for 5 minutes. Season to taste and fluff with a fork.

Meanwhile, heat the oil in a large frying pan, add the vegetables and stir-fry over a moderate heat for 3–4 minutes until piping hot. Cut the preserved lemons into quarters, remove the flesh and discard, then roughly chop the skin.

Stir the vegetables and preserved lemon skin into the couscous with the chickpeas and coriander. Season to taste and serve warm with a spoonful of yogurt and a drizzle of harissa.

....

- **FOR CURRIED VEGETABLE COUSCOUS**

Place 2 teaspoons mild curry paste in a large bowl with 4 tablespoons orange juice and stir together. Add the couscous and 50 g (2 oz) dried cranberries and stir well. Add the boiling water and leave to soak as above. Cook the vegetables as above and stir into the couscous with the chickpeas and coriander. Serve with a spoonful of mango chutney.

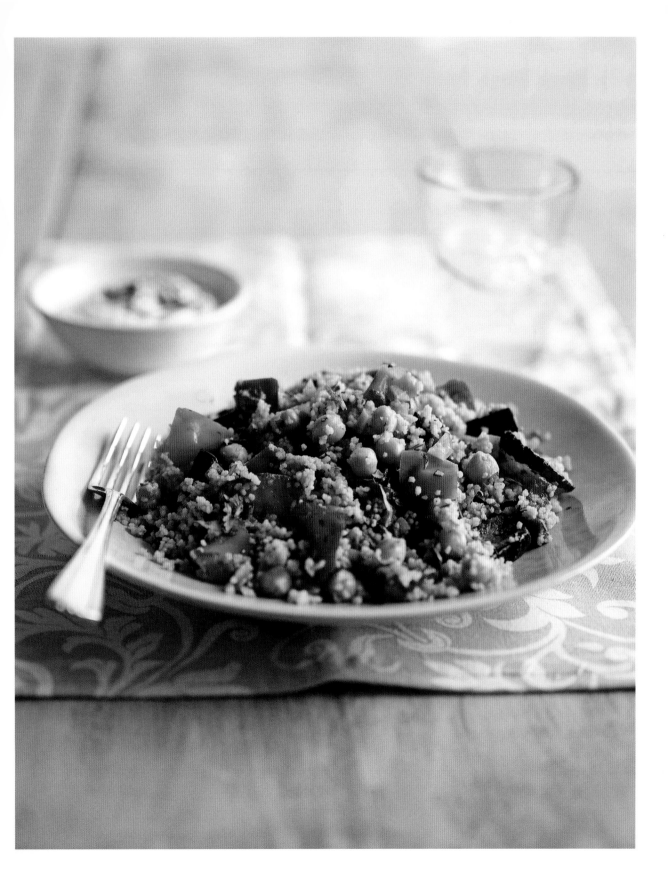

- **SERVES: 4**
- **PREPARATION TIME: 15 MINUTES, PLUS CHILLING**
- **COOKING TIME: 25–30 MINUTES**

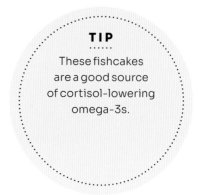

TIP

These fishcakes are a good source of cortisol-lowering omega-3s.

Trout & Dill Fishcakes

300 g (10 oz) trout fillets

400 g (13 oz) mashed potatoes

5 spring onions, finely chopped

2 tablespoons capers, chopped

2 tablespoons chopped dill

grated rind of 1 lemon

2 tablespoons lemon juice

1 tablespoon olive oil

salt and pepper

To serve

steamed Tenderstem broccoli

lime wedges

Cook the trout fillets under a preheated hot grill for 4 minutes on each side until cooked through, then discard the skin, break the flesh into flakes and place in a bowl.

Add the mashed potatoes, spring onions, capers, dill, lemon rind and juice. Season with salt and pepper. Shape into 8 cakes and chill for 20 minutes.

Heat the oil in a frying pan and cook the fishcakes, in batches, for 4–5 minutes on each side or until golden and cooked through. Serve with steamed Tenderstem broccoli and lime wedges.

- **FOR TROUT & DILL PÂTÉ**

Mix together the cooked and flaked trout fillets with 1 teaspoon Dijon mustard, 1 tablespoon chopped dill, 300 g (10 oz) low-fat cream cheese and a pinch of paprika in a bowl. Season to taste. Spoon into 4 ramekins and chill for 30 minutes. Serve with vegetable crudités.

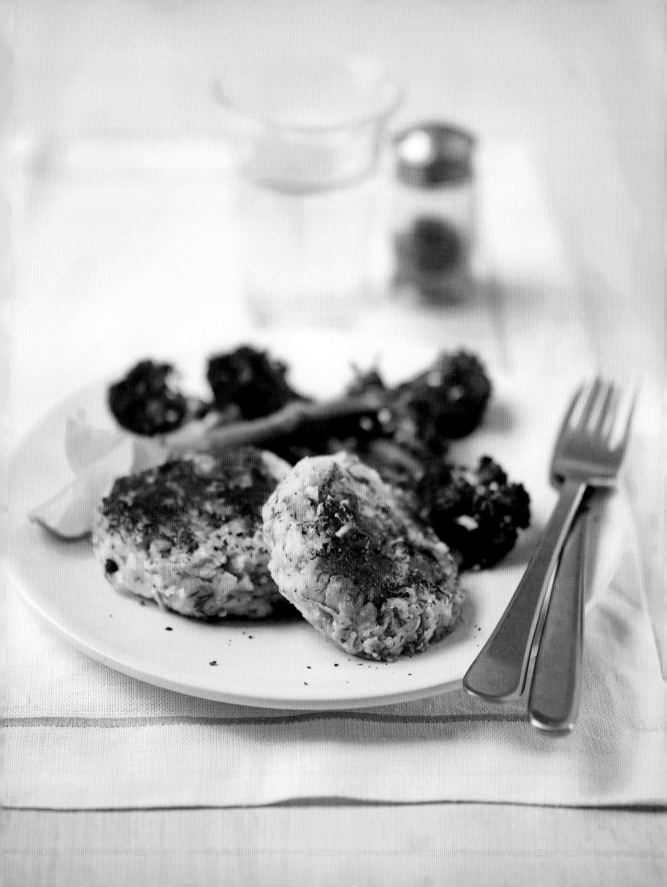

- **SERVES:** 4
- **PREPARATION TIME: 10 MINUTES**
- **COOKING TIME: 40 MINUTES**

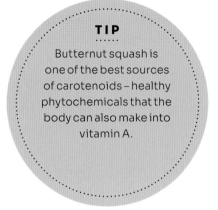

TIP

Butternut squash is one of the best sources of carotenoids – healthy phytochemicals that the body can also make into vitamin A.

Oven-baked Squash with Quinoa

2 tablespoons olive oil

750 g (1½ lb) butternut squash, peeled, deseeded and cut into 3.5 cm (1½ inch) chunks

25 g (1 oz) unsalted butter

1 red onion, chopped

1 garlic clove, crushed

50 g (2 oz) pine nuts

300 g (10 oz) quinoa

150 ml (¼ pint) dry white wine

1 cinnamon stick

1 litre (1¾ pints) vegetable stock

4 tablespoons chopped mint

200 g (7 oz) feta cheese, crumbled

100 g (3½ oz) pomegranate seeds

salt and pepper

Heat the oil in a large frying pan and add the squash in a single layer. Season well with salt and pepper and cook over a medium heat for about 10 minutes until lightly browned.

Meanwhile, melt the butter in a flameproof casserole dish, add the onion and garlic and cook for 2–3 minutes until softened. Stir in the pine nuts and quinoa and cook for 1 minute or until the quinoa is starting to pop. Add the wine and cook until it has been absorbed.

Stir in the squash, cinnamon stick and stock. Bring to the boil, season to taste with salt and pepper and stir well.

Cover the dish with the lid and cook in a preheated oven, 190°C (375°F), Gas Mark 5, for 25 minutes until the quinoa is just tender.

Stir in the mint, then scatter over the feta and pomegranate seeds. Serve immediately.

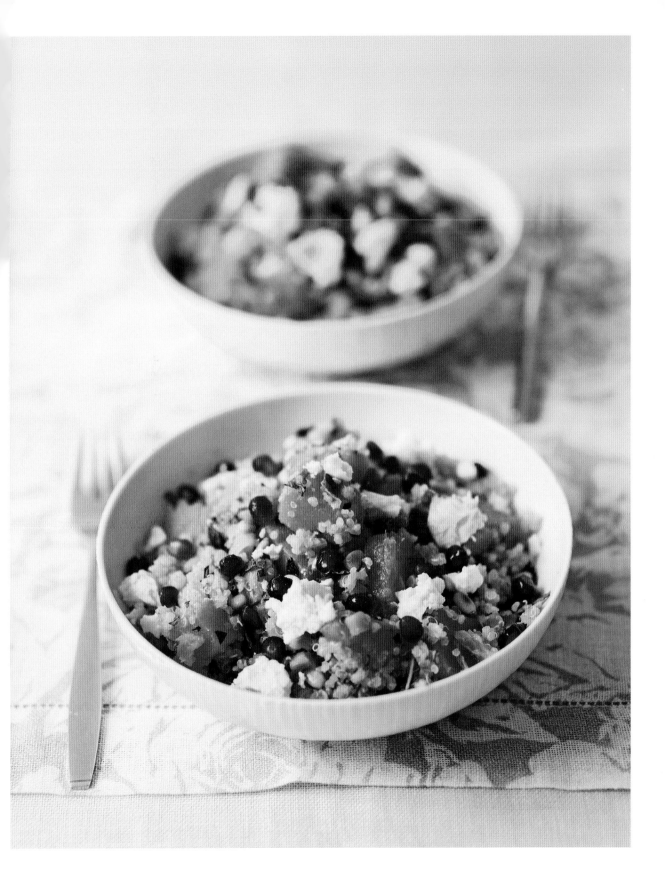

- **SERVES: 4**
- **PREPARATION TIME: 10 MINUTES**
- **COOKING TIME: 20 MINUTES**

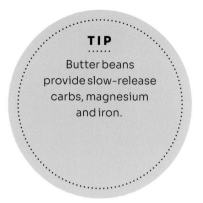

TIP

Butter beans provide slow-release carbs, magnesium and iron.

Butter Bean & Tomato Soup

3 tablespoons olive oil

1 onion, finely chopped

2 celery sticks, thinly sliced

2 garlic cloves, thinly sliced

2 x 400 g (13 oz) cans butter beans, drained

4 tablespoons sun-dried tomato paste

900 ml (1½ pints) vegetable stock

1 tablespoon chopped thyme or rosemary, plus extra leaves to garnish

salt and pepper

Parmesan cheese shavings, to serve

Heat the oil in a saucepan over a medium heat, add the onion and fry for 3 minutes or until softened.

Add the celery and garlic and fry for 2 minutes.

Add the butter beans, sun-dried tomato paste, stock, rosemary or thyme and season with salt and pepper. Bring to the boil, then reduce the heat, cover and simmer gently for 15 minutes.

Ladle into bowls and serve sprinkled with the Parmesan and extra thyme or rosemary leaves. This soup makes a light main course served with bread and plenty of Parmesan.

- **FOR SPICED CARROT & LENTIL SOUP**

Heat 2 tablespoons oil in a saucepan, add 1 chopped onion, 2 crushed garlic cloves and 375 g (12 oz) chopped carrots and fry for 10 minutes. Add a 400 g (13 oz) can lentils, drained, 2 teaspoons ground coriander, 1 teaspoon ground cumin and 1 tablespoon chopped thyme and fry for 1 minute. Stir in 1 litre (1¾ pints) vegetable stock, a 400 g (13 oz) can chopped tomatoes and 2 teaspoons lemon juice and bring to the boil. Cover and simmer gently for 20 minutes. Put in a food processor or blender and blend until smooth, then return to the pan, season to taste and warm through.

- **SERVES: 4**
- **PREPARATION TIME: 5 MINUTES**
- **COOKING TIME: 10 MINUTES**

Chicken & Hummus Wraps

6 skinless chicken thigh fillets,
about 500 g (1 lb) in total

2 tablespoons extra virgin olive oil

grated rind and juice of 1 lemon

1 garlic clove, crushed

1 teaspoon ground cumin

4 wholewheat flour tortillas

200 g (7 oz) hummus

25 g (1 oz) wild rocket leaves

handful of parsley leaves

salt and pepper

Cut the chicken thighs into quarters and put in a bowl. Combine the oil, lemon rind, garlic, cumin and salt and pepper to taste, add to the chicken and stir well.

Heat a ridged griddle pan until hot. Thread the chicken pieces on to metal skewers, place in the pan and cook for 4–5 minutes on each side until cooked through. Remove and leave to rest for 5 minutes.

Meanwhile, warm the tortillas in a preheated oven, 150°C (350°F), Gas Mark 2, for 5 minutes.

Remove the chicken from the skewers. Divide the hummus, rocket leaves, parsley and chicken between the tortillas. Squeeze over the lemon juice, wrap and serve.

- **FOR EASY HOMEMADE HUMMUS**

Put 400 g (13 oz) can chickpeas (drained), 1 crushed garlic clove, 3 tablespoons extra virgin olive oil, 1 tablespoon lemon juice and salt and pepper to taste in a food processor or blender and process until smooth.

- **SERVES: 4**
- **PREPARATION TIME: 15 MINUTES**
- **COOKING TIME: 10–12 MINUTES**

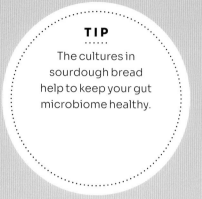

TIP

The cultures in sourdough bread help to keep your gut microbiome healthy.

Aubergine Toasties with Pesto

1 large aubergine

4 tablespoons extra virgin olive oil

4 slices of sourdough bread

2 beefsteak tomatoes, thickly sliced

200 g (7 oz) mozzarella cheese, sliced

salt and pepper

Pesto

50 g (2 oz) basil leaves

1 garlic clove, crushed

4 tablespoons pine nuts

100 ml (3½ fl oz) extra virgin olive oil

2 tablespoons freshly grated Parmesan cheese

First make the pesto. Put the basil, garlic, pine nuts, oil and salt and pepper in a food processor and process until fairly smooth. Transfer to a bowl, stir in the Parmesan and adjust the seasoning. Set aside until required.

Cut the aubergines into 1 cm (½ inch) thick slices. Season the oil with salt and pepper and brush over the aubergine slices. Heat a ridged griddle pan until hot. Add the aubergine slices, in batches if necessary, and cook for 4–5 minutes on each side until charred and tender.

Meanwhile, grill the sourdough bread.

Top the grilled bread with aubergine slices. Spread with the pesto. Top with tomato and mozzarella slices and more pesto. Cook under a preheated hot grill for 1–2 minutes until bubbling and golden.

- **FOR AUBERGINE BUCK RAREBIT**

Arrange the cooked aubergine slices on large toasted soft bread roll halves with the pesto, sliced tomatoes and mozzarella. Grill until brown. Top each with a poached egg and serve immediately.

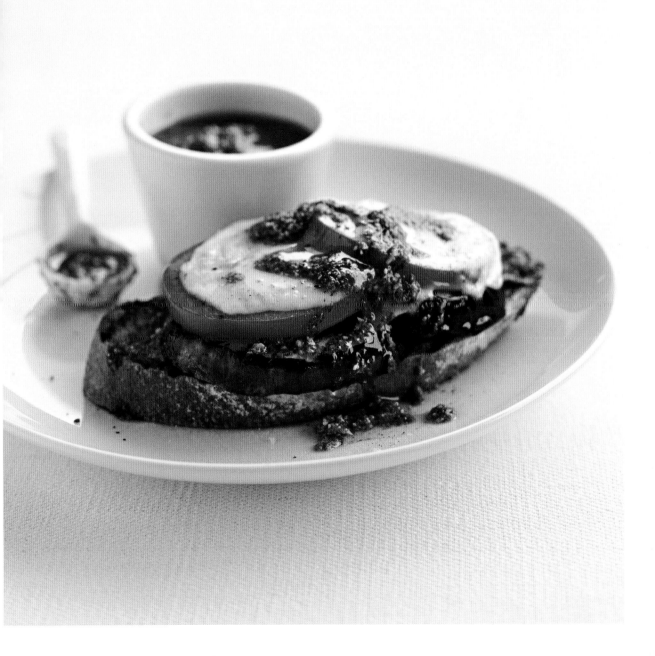

- **SERVES: 4**
- **PREPARATION TIME: 15 MINUTES, PLUS SOAKING**
- **COOKING TIME: 12 MINUTES**

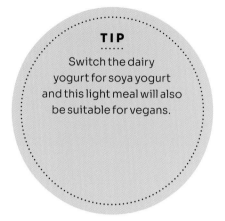

TIP

Switch the dairy yogurt for soya yogurt and this light meal will also be suitable for vegans.

Falafel Pitta Pockets

250 g (8 oz) dried chickpeas

1 small onion, finely chopped

2 garlic cloves, crushed

½ bunch of parsley

½ bunch of coriander

2 teaspoons ground coriander

½ teaspoon baking powder

vegetable oil, for shallow frying

4 wholemeal pitta breads

handful of salad leaves

2 tomatoes, diced

4 tablespoons fat-free Greek yogurt

salt and pepper

Put the chickpeas in a bowl, add cold water to cover by a generous 10 cm (4 inches) and leave to soak overnight.

Drain the chickpeas, transfer to a food processor and process until coarsely ground. Add the onion, garlic, herbs, ground coriander and baking powder. Season with salt and pepper and process until really smooth. Using wet hands, shape the mixture into 16 small patties.

Heat a little vegetable oil in a large frying pan over a medium-high heat, add the patties, in batches, and fry for 3 minutes on each side or until golden and cooked through. Remove with a slotted spoon and drain on kitchen paper.

Split the pitta breads and fill with the falafel, salad leaves and diced tomatoes. Add a spoonful of the yogurt to each and serve immediately.

- **FOR FALAFEL SALAD**

Toss 4 handfuls of mixed salad leaves with a little olive oil, lemon juice and salt and pepper and arrange on serving plates. Core, deseed and dice 1 red pepper and sprinkle it over the salads. Top with the cooked falafel and spoon over a little yogurt.

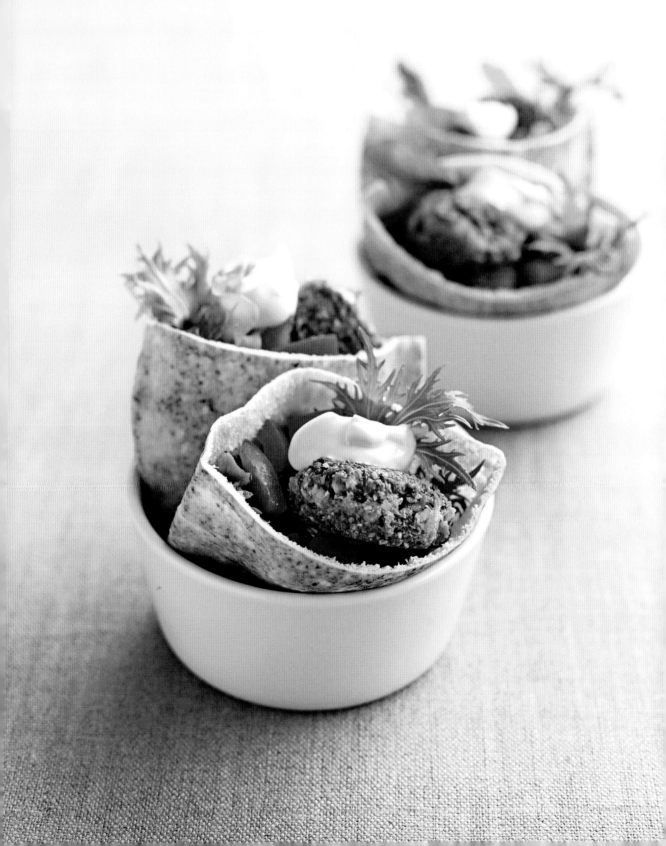

- **SERVES: 4**
- **PREPARATION TIME: 10 MINUTES**
- **COOKING TIME: 15 MINUTES**

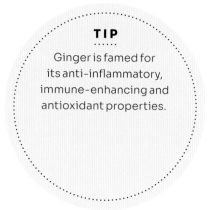

TIP

Ginger is famed for its anti-inflammatory, immune-enhancing and antioxidant properties.

Ginger Chicken Soup

1 tablespoon groundnut oil

2.5 cm (1 inch) piece of fresh root ginger, peeled and grated

300 g (10 oz) chicken breast fillets, cut into strips

1 litre (1¾ pints) hot chicken stock

4 pak choi, sliced

175 g (6 oz) dried egg noodles

2 tablespoons sesame seeds

Heat the oil in a wok or large saucepan, add the ginger and stir-fry for 1 minute, then stir in the chicken and 125 ml (4 fl oz) of the stock. Bring to the boil, then cook over a high heat for 5 minutes or until the chicken is cooked through.

Add the remaining stock and bring to a simmer. Stir in the pak choi and noodles and simmer for 5 minutes until the noodles are cooked.

Meanwhile, heat a nonstick frying pan over a medium-low heat and dry-fry the sesame seeds for 2 minutes, stirring frequently, until golden brown and toasted.

Ladle the soup into bowls and serve sprinkled with the toasted sesame seeds.

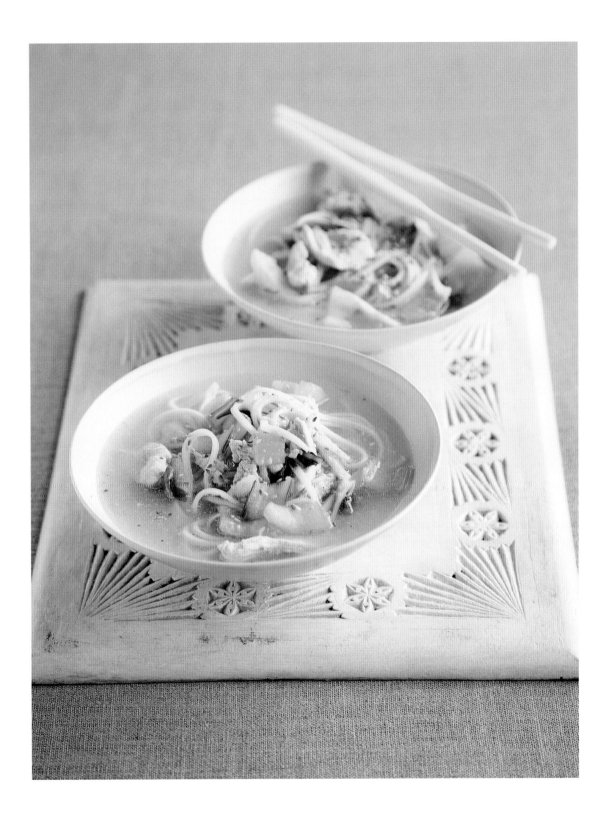

- **SERVES: 4**
- **PREPARATION TIME: 10 MINUTES**
- **COOKING TIME: 20 MINUTES**

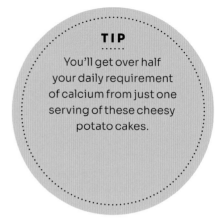

Cheese & Paprika Potato Cakes

750 g (1½ lb) small equal-sized potatoes

225 g (7½ oz) hard, tangy sheep's or mature Cheddar cheese, finely diced

1–2 teaspoons cumin seeds

2 teaspoons smoked paprika

4 tablespoons plain flour

sunflower or vegetable oil, for shallow frying

salt and pepper

chopped parsley, to garnish

lemon wedges, to serve

Cook the potatoes in a saucepan of boiling water for 10–12 minutes until soft. Drain, then refresh under cold running water and peel off the skins. Place in a bowl and roughly mash with a fork until still a little chunky. Add the cheese, cumin seeds and paprika and season.

Tip the flour onto a plate. Divide the potato mixture into 12 pieces, shape each piece into a ball, then flatten slightly and dip into the flour to lightly coat on both sides.

Heat a thin layer of oil in a large, heavy-based frying pan, add the potato cakes and cook for about 8 minutes, turning occasionally, until crispy and golden brown. Drain on kitchen paper, sprinkle with a little extra sea salt, garnish with chopped parsley and serve with lemon wedges.

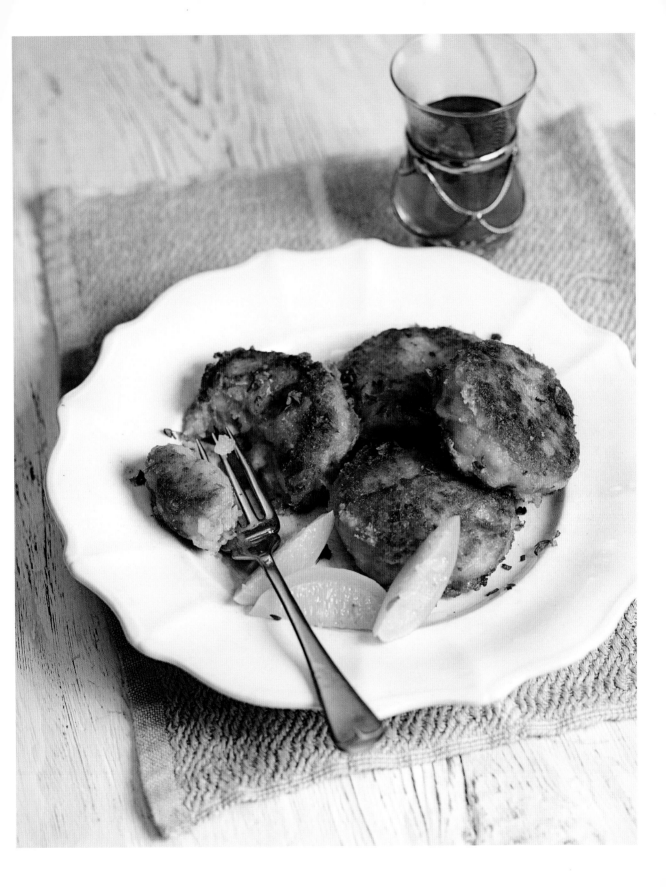

- **SERVES:** 4
- **PREPARATION TIME:** 15 MINUTES, PLUS COOLING
- **COOKING TIME:** ABOUT 15 MINUTES

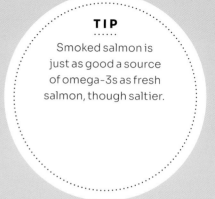

TIP

Smoked salmon is just as good a source of omega-3s as fresh salmon, though saltier.

Salmon & Cucumber Sushi

300 g (10 oz) sushi rice

2 tablespoons rice vinegar

1 tablespoon caster sugar

2 nori sheets

1 teaspoon wasabi paste

4 long strips of cucumber, the length of the nori and about 1 cm (½ inch) thick

100 g (3½ oz) smoked salmon

2 tablespoons pickled ginger

4 tablespoons soy sauce

Cook the sushi rice according to the packet instructions.

Mix together the vinegar and sugar in a bowl and stir until the sugar dissolves. Once the rice is cooked, and when it is still warm, mix in enough of the vinegar and sugar mixture to coat the rice grains, but do not allow the rice to become wet. Tip the rice on to a tray to cool quickly.

Take 1 nori sheet and place it on a bamboo mat with the longest side in line with your body and the ridged surface facing upwards. With damp hands, cover three-quarters of the nori sheet with a thin layer of rice, leaving a band of nori at the top without rice.

Spread a little wasabi paste with your finger on top of the rice in a thin line, at the edge nearest to you. Then place 2 cucumber strips and half the smoked salmon on the wasabi.

Use the bamboo mat to start rolling the nori up, tucking in the cucumber and salmon as you go. Once you have rolled up the majority of the nori, wet your finger and dampen the plain edge of nori. Finish rolling up the nori. The wet edge will stick the roll together. Repeat with the other nori sheet. Then, using a sharp knife, cut the rolls into 8 even pieces or 4 even pieces and 1 slightly larger piece cut into 2 on the diagonal.

Mix the remaining wasabi and soy sauce and serve with the pickled ginger alongside the nori rolls.

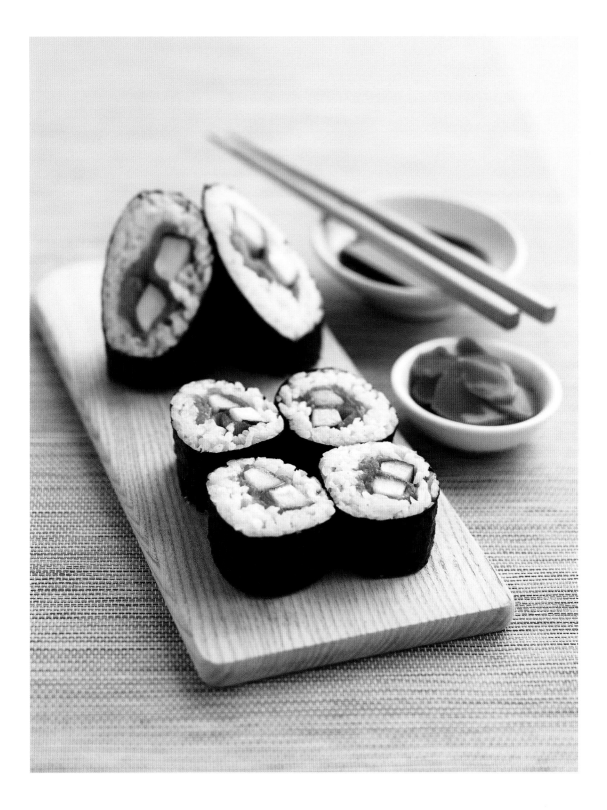

- **SERVES: 4–6**
- **PREPARATION TIME: 10 MINUTES**
- **COOKING TIME: 35 MINUTES**

TIP

These colourful vegetables contain carotenoids, a group of healthy, fat-soluble phytochemicals that are better absorbed when cooked in oil.

Braised Vegetables

5 tablespoons olive oil

1 onion, sliced

2 garlic cloves, sliced

200 g (7 oz) can chopped tomatoes

1 green pepper, cored, deseeded and sliced

1 aubergine or 3 baby aubergines, sliced

1 courgette or 4 baby courgettes, sliced

salt and pepper

Heat 1 tablespoon of the oil in a large frying pan over a medium heat, add the onion and cook for 5–7 minutes until softened. Stir in the garlic and cook for a further 1 minute. Add the tomatoes and a little water and simmer for 15 minutes.

Meanwhile, heat 1 tablespoon of the oil in a separate frying pan, add the green pepper and cook for 5 minutes, stirring, until softened and lightly browned. Remove from the pan and set aside. Add another 2 tablespoons of the oil to the pan, add the aubergine and cook for 5 minutes until golden, then set aside. Add the remaining oil to the pan, add the courgette and cook for 5 minutes until golden.

Return the pepper and aubergine to the pan, pour over the tomato sauce and season well. Bring to the boil, then reduce the heat and simmer for 10 minutes until the vegetables are very tender and most of the liquid has evaporated.

- **FOR SUMMERY VEGETABLE FLATBREADS**

Prepare the braised vegetables as above and leave to cool. Using a 150 g (5 oz) packet pizza base mix, make the dough according to the packet instructions. Divide into 4 pieces, then roll out each piece on a lightly floured work surface to an oval shape and place on lightly greased baking sheets. Spoon over the braised vegetables and bake in a preheated oven, 200°C (400°F), Gas Mark 6, for 15–20 minutes until the bases are crisp.

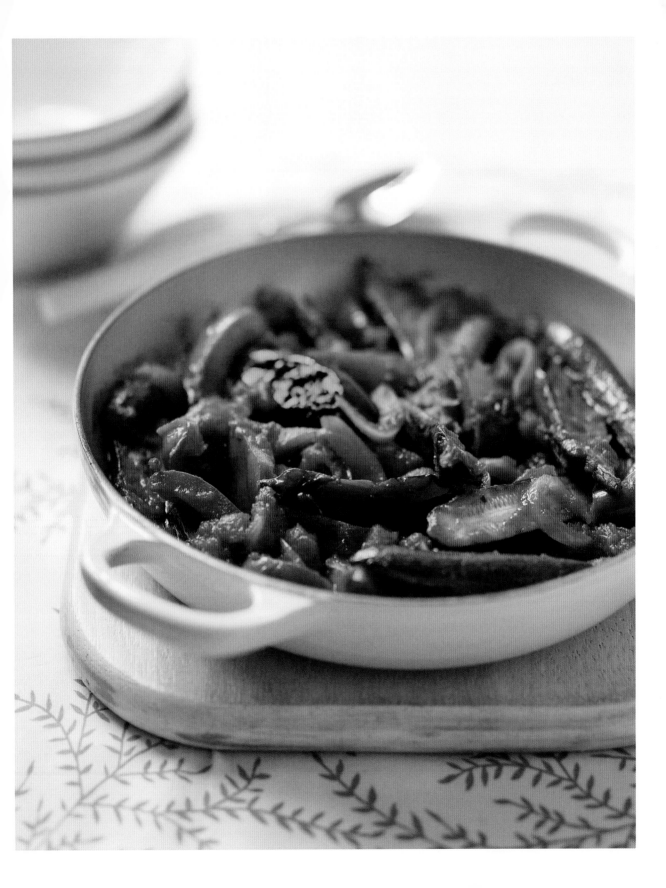

- **SERVES: 2**
- **PREPARATION TIME: 10 MINUTES**
- **COOKING TIME: 1 HOUR**

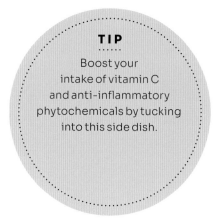

TIP

Boost your intake of vitamin C and anti-inflammatory phytochemicals by tucking into this side dish.

Roasted Stuffed Peppers

4 large red peppers, halved lengthways, cored and deseeded

2 garlic cloves, crushed

1 tablespoon chopped thyme, plus extra to garnish

4 plum tomatoes, halved

4 tablespoons extra virgin olive oil

2 tablespoons balsamic vinegar

salt and pepper

To serve

crusty bread (optional)

baby leaf salad (optional)

Place the pepper halves, cut sides up, in an ovenproof dish or a roasting tin lined with foil. Divide the garlic and thyme between them and season with salt and pepper.

Put a tomato half in each pepper. Drizzle with the oil and vinegar. Roast in a preheated oven, 220°C (425°F), Gas Mark 7, for about 1 hour until the peppers are soft and charred.

Serve with some crusty bread to mop up the juices and a baby leaf salad, if liked.

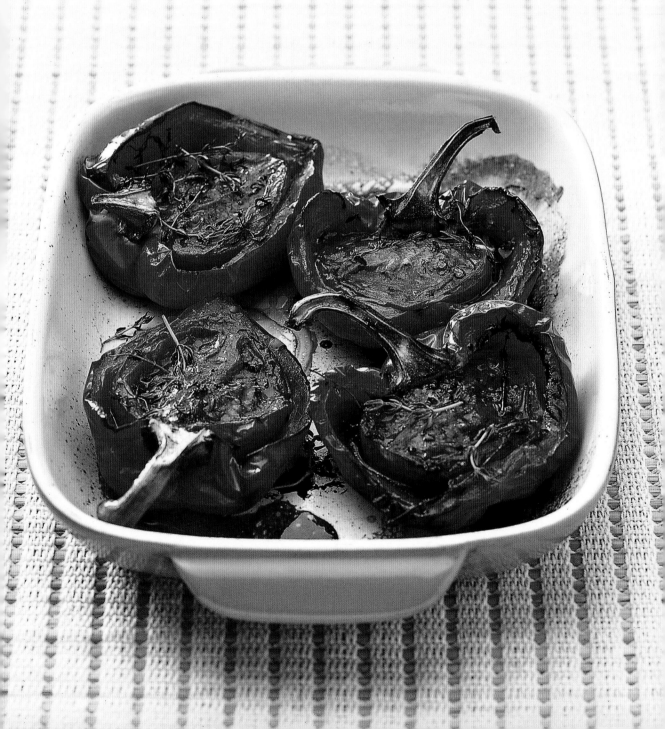

- **SERVES: 4**
- **PREPARATION TIME: 15 MINUTES**
- **COOKING TIME: 20–25 MINUTES**

Pumpkin with Walnut Pesto

1 kg (2 lb) pumpkin

extra virgin olive oil, for brushing

salt and pepper

Walnut pesto

50 g (2 oz) walnuts, toasted

2 spring onions, chopped

1 large garlic clove, crushed

50 g (2 oz) rocket leaves, plus extra to serve

3 tablespoons walnut oil

3 tablespoons extra virgin olive oil

Cut the pumpkin into 8 wedges. Remove the seeds and fibre but leave the skin on. Brush all over with olive oil, season with salt and pepper and spread out on a large baking sheet. Roast in a preheated oven, 220°C (425°F), Gas Mark 7, for 20–25 minutes until tender, turning halfway through.

Meanwhile, make the pesto. Put the walnuts, spring onions, garlic and rocket in a food processor and process until finely chopped. With the motor running, gradually drizzle in the oils. Season the pesto with salt and pepper.

Serve the roasted pumpkin with the pesto and extra rocket leaves.

- **FOR GNOCCHI WITH WALNUT PESTO**

Make the pesto as above. Cook 500 g (1 lb) ready-made gnocchi in a large saucepan of lightly salted boiling water for 5–6 minutes until the gnocchi rise to the surface, then drain, transfer to a buttered serving dish and top with the pesto.

- **SERVES: 4**
- **PREPARATION TIME: 10 MINUTES, PLUS STANDING**
- **COOKING TIME: 5 MINUTES**

Green Beans with Almonds

1 teaspoon Dijon mustard

2 tablespoons white wine vinegar

1 shallot, finely chopped

3 tablespoons olive oil

500 g (1 lb) green beans

2 tablespoons toasted
slivered almonds

Mix together the mustard and vinegar in a bowl. Add the shallot, leave to stand for 10 minutes, then whisk in the oil.

Trim and blanch the beans in a saucepan of lightly salted boiling water until just tender, then toss them in the dressing and serve in a salad bowl topped with the slivered almonds.

- **FOR GREEN BEANS WITH ANCHOVY DRESSING**

Put 150 ml (¼ pint) olive oil into a small, heavy-based saucepan and add 3 canned anchovies. Cook over a low heat for 5 minutes until the anchovies have softened and broken down. Remove the pan from the heat and leave to cool to room temperature. Whisk in 2 tablespoons white wine vinegar and some cracked black pepper. Cook the green beans as above, toss in the dressing and serve immediately.

- **SERVES: 4**
- **PREPARATION TIME: 20 MINUTES**
- **COOKING TIME: 15 MINUTES**

Aubergine with Caper & Mint Dressing

2 aubergines, trimmed and sliced

150 ml (¼ pint) extra virgin olive oil

warm pitta bread, to serve

Dressing

finely grated rind and juice of 1 lemon

3 tablespoons olive oil

2 tablespoons red wine vinegar

4 tablespoons chopped mint leaves, plus extra leaves to garnish

2 tablespoons capers, roughly chopped

1 garlic clove, roughly chopped

1 teaspooon sugar

salt and pepper

Put the aubergine slices in a large bowl, pour over the oil and toss well to coat evenly. The oil will be absorbed fast, so work as quickly as possible. Set aside for 10 minutes while making the dressing.

Mix all the dressing ingredients together in a jug. Season with a little salt and pepper.

Heat a griddle pan until smoking, then lay several of the aubergine slices on to the hot pan in a single layer and cook over a high heat for 1–2 minutes on each side until lightly charred and soft. Transfer to a heatproof platter and keep warm in a low oven while cooking the remaining slices.

Drizzle or spoon some of the dressing over the aubergine slices, garnish with extra mint leaves and serve with warm pitta bread, with the remaining dressing in a jug.

- **FOR WARM GRIDDLED VEGETABLES WITH BASIL DRESSING**

Cut 2 red peppers into quarters, discarding the cores and seeds, and put in a bowl. Add 2 courgettes, trimmed and sliced lengthways, and 4 large mushrooms, trimmed, then pour over 6 tablespoons olive oil and toss well. To make the dressing, mix together 4 tablespoons chopped basil, 3 tablespoons olive oil and 2 tablespoons each red wine vinegar and lightly toasted pine nuts, roughly chopped, in a jug. Season generously with salt and pepper. Heat a griddle pan until smoking, add the vegetables, in batches, and cook over a high heat for 2–3 minutes on each side until lightly charred and soft. Arrange on a serving platter and drizzle with the dressing to serve.

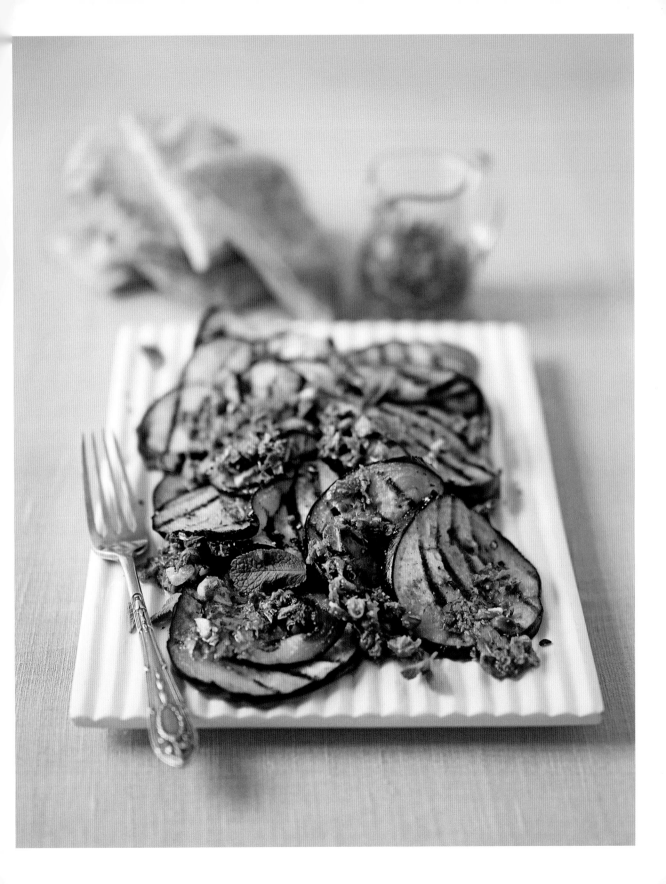

- **SERVES: 4**
- **PREPARATION TIME: 10 MINUTES**
- **COOKING TIME: 25–35 MINUTES**

Spicy Roasted Cherry Tomatoes

450 g (14½ oz) cherry tomatoes

2 tablespoons olive oil

4 garlic cloves, halved and smashed

1–2 teaspoons finely chopped dried red chillies

1 teaspoon sugar

finely chopped rind of ½ preserved lemon

salt

crusty bread, to serve (optional)

Put the tomatoes in a roasting tin, drizzle over the oil, scatter the garlic, chillies and sugar over the tomatoes and toss to coat well.

Place, uncovered, in a preheated oven, 200°C (400°F), Gas Mark 6, for 20–25 minutes until the tomato skins begin to wrinkle.

Sprinkle the preserved lemon rind over the tomatoes and stir to coat well, then season with salt. Return to the oven for 5–10 minutes. Serve with chunks of crusty bread or as an accompaniment to grilled and roasted dishes.

- **FOR ROASTED CHERRY TOMATOES WITH FETA & MINT**

Put 450 g (14½ oz) cherry tomatoes in a roasting tin, drizzle over 2 tablespoons olive oil, scatter over 4 garlic cloves, halved and smashed, and 1 teaspoon sugar and toss to coat well. Place, uncovered, in a preheated oven, 200°C (400°F), Gas Mark 6, for 20–25 minutes, then toss in 1–2 teaspoons dried mint and scatter 150 g (5 oz) crumbled feta cheese over the top. Return to the oven for 5–10 minutes. Garnish with 1 tablespoon finely chopped mint.

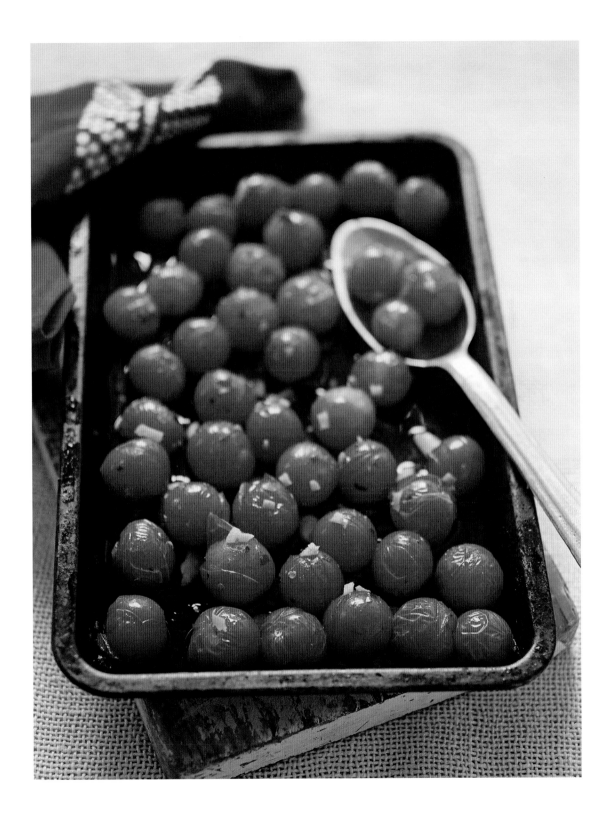

- **SERVES: 4–6**
- **PREPARATION TIME: 10 MINUTES, PLUS SOAKING**
- **COOKING TIME: 1¼ HOURS**

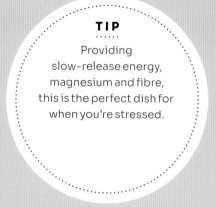

TIP
Providing slow-release energy, magnesium and fibre, this is the perfect dish for when you're stressed.

Beans & Peppers with Harissa

225 g (7½ oz) dried butter beans, soaked in water overnight

225 g (7½ oz) dried kidney beans, soaked in water overnight

2 tablespoons olive oil

knob of butter

2 onions, finely chopped

4–6 garlic cloves, smashed

2 teaspoons sugar

2 teaspoons cumin seeds

2 red, orange or yellow peppers, cored, deseeded and diced

1–2 teaspoons harissa paste

2 x 400 g (13 oz) cans chopped tomatoes

small bunch of mint, finely chopped

salt and pepper

To serve

chunks of bread (optional)

natural yogurt (optional)

Drain and rinse the butter and kidney beans. Place them in a large saucepan filled with water. Bring to the boil, then reduce the heat and simmer for about 40 minutes until tender. Drain and refresh under cold running water, then remove any loose skins.

Heat the oil and butter in a large, heavy-based saucepan over a medium heat, stir in the onions, garlic and sugar and cook for 2–3 minutes to soften. Add the cumin seeds and peppers and cook for a further 1–2 minutes, then add the drained beans and stir to coat well.

Stir in the harissa and the tomatoes and cook over a gentle heat for 30 minutes. Season to taste with salt and pepper, then stir in half the mint and garnish with the remaining mint. Serve with chunks of bread and a dollop of creamy yogurt, if liked.

- **FOR BEANS WITH MINT & FETA**

Follow the recipe above, omitting the peppers, harissa and tomatoes, adding 1–2 teaspoons dried mint and the juice of 1 lemon instead. Cover and cook gently for 10–15 minutes, then stir in the chopped fresh mint, crumble 150 g (5 oz) feta cheese over the top, and serve with toasted flatbreads.

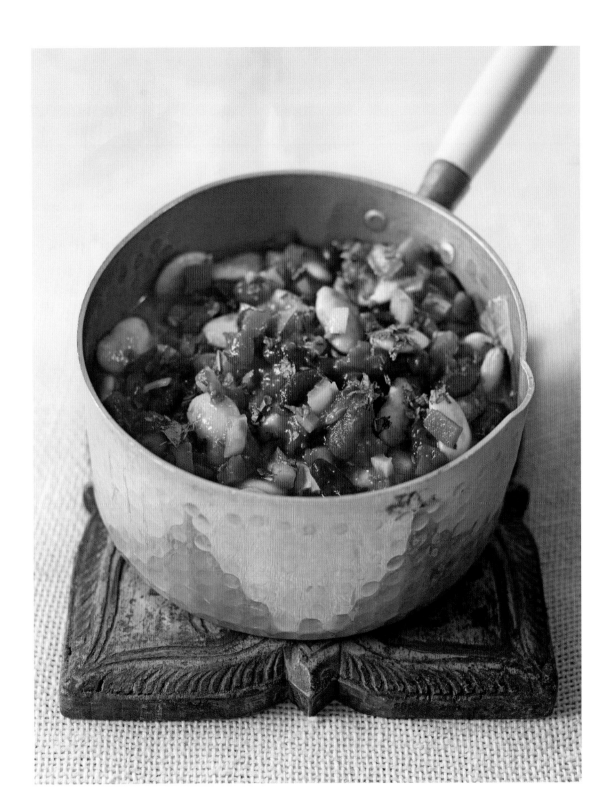

- **SERVES: 4**
- **PREPARATION TIME: 20 MINUTES**
- **COOKING TIME: ABOUT 35 MINUTES**

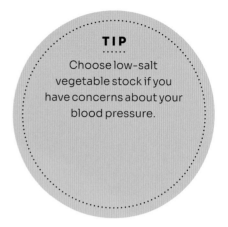

TIP

Choose low-salt vegetable stock if you have concerns about your blood pressure.

Baked Carrot & Potato Tagine

2–3 tablespoons olive oil

2 onions, thickly sliced

4 garlic cloves, finely chopped

25 g (1 oz) fresh root ginger, peeled and finely chopped

1–2 red chillies, deseeded and finely chopped

2 teaspoons cumin seeds

1 teaspoon fennel seeds

4 large potatoes, peeled and thickly sliced

2 large carrots, peeled and thickly sliced

300 ml (½ pint) vegetable or chicken stock

finely sliced rind of 1 preserved lemon

3–4 tomatoes, sliced

15 g (½ oz) butter, cut into small pieces

salt and pepper

coriander, finely chopped, to garnish

couscous, to serve (optional)

Heat the oil in a heavy-based saucepan over a medium heat, stir in the onions and cook for 1–2 minutes until they begin to soften. Add the garlic, ginger, chillies, cumin and fennel seeds and cook for a further 1–2 minutes.

Add the potatoes and carrots and pour in the stock. Bring to the boil, then reduce the heat, cover and cook gently for 15 minutes. Transfer the vegetables to a tagine or ovenproof dish.

Stir in the preserved lemon rind, season with salt and pepper and arrange the tomato slices over the top. Dot the tomatoes with the butter, then place, uncovered, in a preheated oven, 180°C (350°F), Gas Mark 4, for 15 minutes until the tomatoes are lightly browned. Garnish with coriander and serve with couscous, if liked.

- **FOR BAKED POTATO & TOMATO TAGINE**

Make the tagine as above, omitting the fennel seeds and carrots, adding 150 g (5 oz) crumbled feta cheese with the preserved lemon and increasing the quantity of potatoes to 6.

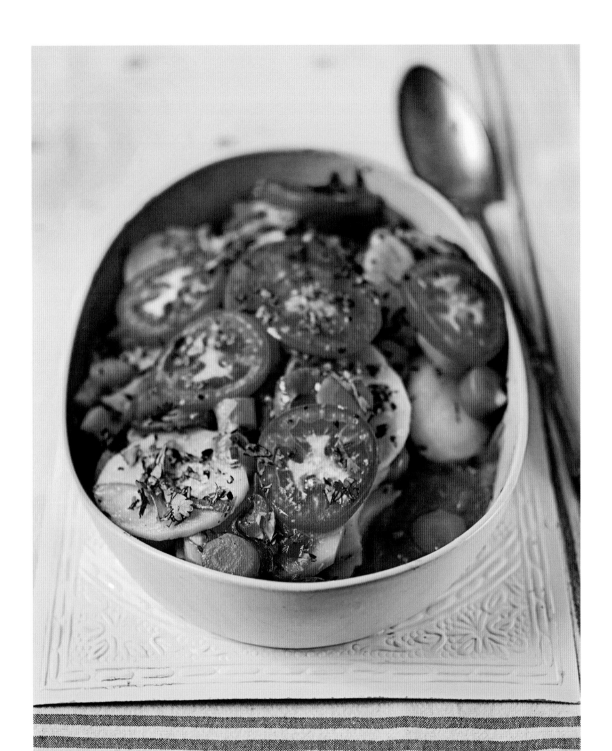

- **SERVES: 4**
- **PREPARATION TIME: 15 MINUTES**
- **COOKING TIME: 30–35 MINUTES**

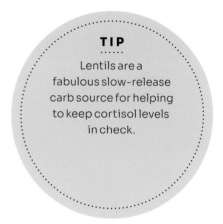

TIP

Lentils are a fabulous slow-release carb source for helping to keep cortisol levels in check.

Lentils with Celery & Carrots

2 tablespoons olive oil

1–2 teaspoons caraway seeds

4 garlic cloves, finely chopped

1 chilli, deseeded and finely chopped

2 carrots, peeled and diced

2 celery sticks, trimmed and diced

175 g (6 oz) dried brown lentils, rinsed and drained

600 ml (1 pint) chicken or vegetable stock

small bunch of flat leaf parsley, finely chopped

salt and pepper

1 lemon, cut into wedges, to serve

Heat the oil in a large, heavy-based saucepan over a medium heat, stir in the caraway seeds, garlic and chilli and cook for 1–2 minutes to let the flavours mingle. Add the carrots and celery, stir to coat well and cook for a further 1–2 minutes, then add the lentils.

Pour in the stock and bring to the boil, then reduce the heat, cover and cook gently for 25–30 minutes until the lentils are tender but not mushy. Season to taste with salt and pepper, then stir in the parsley. Serve as a side dish with wedges of lemon to squeeze over.

- **FOR LENTILS WITH CELERY & HARISSA**

Heat the oil in a large, heavy-based saucepan, stir in 2 finely chopped garlic cloves and cook for 1–2 minutes. Trim and dice 2 celery sticks and add them to the garlic. Stir in 1–2 teaspoons harissa paste, then add 225 g (7½ oz) rinsed and drained brown lentils and pour in 600 ml (1 pint) water. Bring to the boil, reduce the heat, cover and cook gently for 25–30 minutes. Season and serve as above.

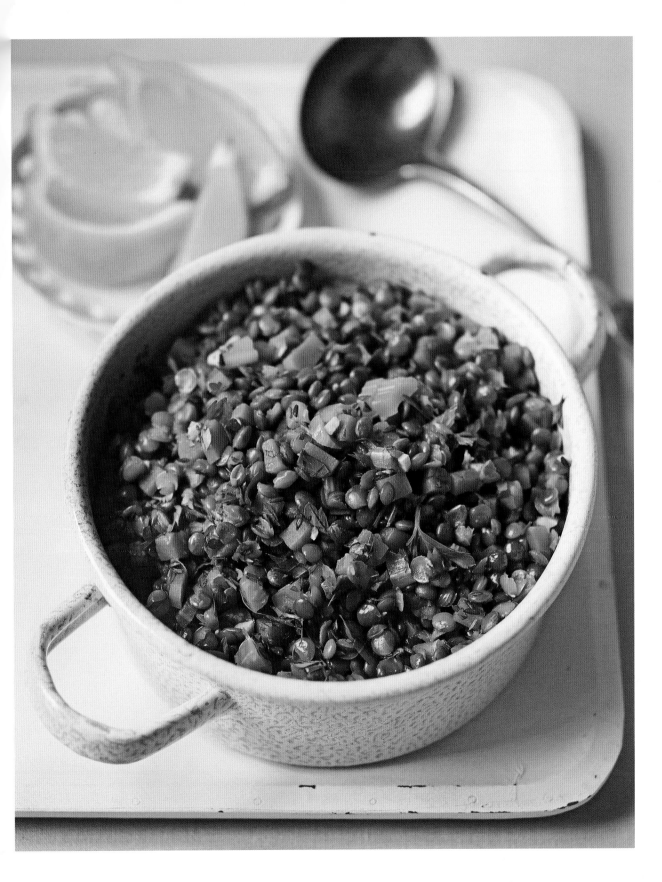

Something Sweet

- **SERVES: 6**
- **PREPARATION TIME: 20 MINUTES, PLUS COOLING**
- **COOKING TIME: 30 MINUTES**

Pistachio Chocolate Brownies

200 g (7 oz) plain dark chocolate, broken into pieces

200 g (7 oz) butter, diced

200 g (7 oz) light muscovado sugar

3 eggs

50 g (2 oz) plain flour

1 teaspoon baking powder

50 g (2 oz) pistachio nuts, roughly chopped

vanilla ice cream, to serve

Sauce

100 g (3½ oz) plain dark chocolate, broken into pieces

150 ml (¼ pint) semi-skimmed milk

2 tablespoons light muscovado sugar

Line a 20 cm (8 inch) square cake tin with nonstick baking paper.

Melt the chocolate and butter together in a heatproof bowl set over a saucepan of gently simmering water, stirring occasionally, making sure that the water doesn't touch the base of the bowl.

Whisk the sugar and eggs together in a large bowl with a hand-held electric whisk until pale, very thick and the whisk leaves a trail when lifted out of the mixture. Fold in the melted chocolate mixture, then the flour and baking powder.

Pour the mixture into the prepared tin and sprinkle with the pistachios. Bake in a preheated oven, 180°C (350°F), Gas Mark 4, for about 25 minutes until the top is crusty but the centre is still slightly soft. Leave to cool and harden in the tin.

Make the sauce. Heat all the sauce ingredients together gently in a saucepan, stirring until smooth.

Lift the brownies out of the tin using the paper. Cut into small squares, lift off the paper and transfer to serving plates. Add scoops of vanilla ice cream and serve with the warm chocolate sauce.

- **FOR WHITE CHOCOLATE & CRANBERRY BLONDIES**

Melt 200 g (7 oz) white chocolate, broken into pieces, with 125 g (4 oz) diced butter as above. Whisk 150 g (5 oz) caster sugar with 3 eggs as above, then fold in the melted chocolate mixture. Fold in 150 g (5 oz) self-raising flour and 50 g (2 oz) dried cranberries. Bake as above.

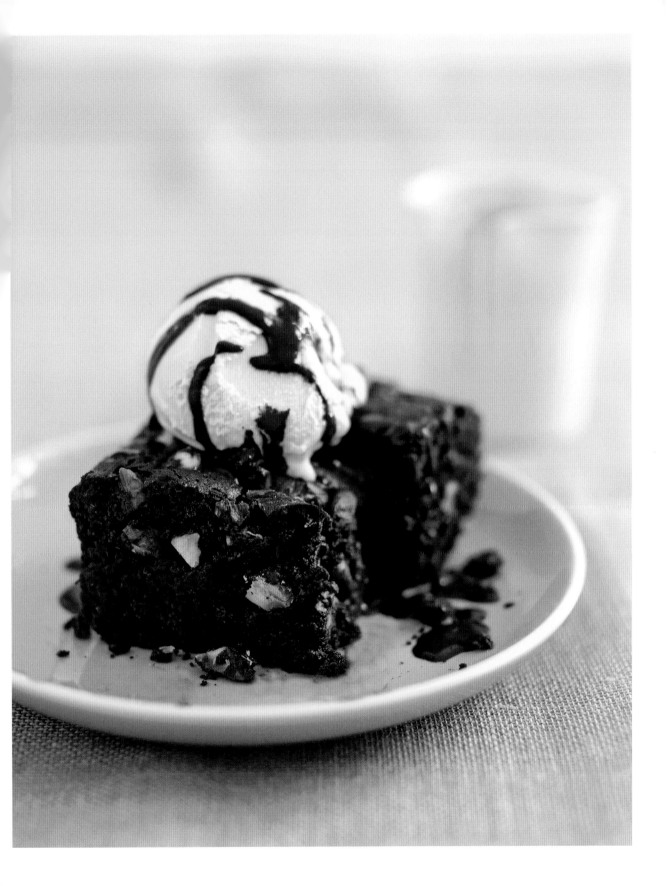

- **SERVES: 4**
- **PREPARATION TIME: 10 MINUTES**
- **COOKING TIME: 25 MINUTES**

TIP

This pud counts as at least one of your daily fruit portions and is a great source of fibre, too!

Rhubarb & Raspberry Crumble

500 g (1 lb) fresh or defrosted frozen rhubarb, sliced

125 g (4 oz) fresh or frozen raspberries

50 g (2 oz) soft light brown sugar

3 tablespoons orange juice

low-fat crème fraîche, to serve

Crumble topping

200 g (7 oz) wholemeal plain flour

pinch of salt

150 g (5 oz) unsalted butter

200 g (7 oz) soft light brown sugar

Make the crumble topping. Combine the flour and salt in a bowl, add the butter and rub in with the fingertips until the mixture resembles breadcrumbs. Stir in the sugar.

Mix the fruits, the sugar and orange juice together in a separate bowl, then tip into a greased ovenproof dish. Sprinkle over the topping and bake in a preheated oven, 200°C (400°F), Gas Mark 6, for about 25 minutes or until golden brown and bubbling.

Serve the crumble hot with low-fat crème fraîche.

- **FOR APPLE & BLACKBERRY CRUMBLE**

Follow the recipe above, using 450 g (14½ oz) each of apples, peeled and chopped, and fresh or frozen blackberries in place of the rhubarb and raspberries. Alternatively, you could use 450 g (14½ oz) plums, stoned and quartered, and 4 peeled, cored and thinly sliced ripe pears.

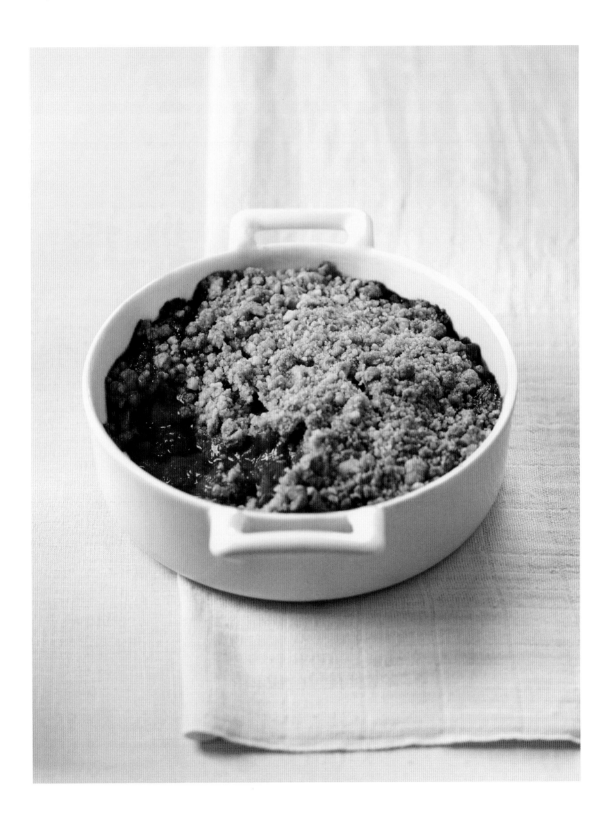

- SERVES: 4
- PREPARATION TIME: 5 MINUTES
- COOKING TIME: 8–10 MINUTES

TIP

Bananas contain prebiotics which feed your good gut bacteria. Slightly less ripe bananas have more prebiotics than overripe ones.

Griddled Bananas with Blueberries

4 bananas, unpeeled

8 tablespoons fat-free Greek yogurt

4 tablespoons oatmeal or fine porridge oats

125 g (4 oz) blueberries

runny honey, to serve

Heat a ridged griddle pan over a medium-hot heat, add the bananas and griddle for 8–10 minutes, or until the skins are beginning to blacken, turning occasionally.

Transfer the bananas to serving dishes and, using a sharp knife, cut open lengthways. Spoon over the yogurt and sprinkle with the oatmeal or oats and blueberries. Serve immediately, drizzled with a little honey.

- **FOR OATMEAL, GINGER & SULTANA YOGURT**

Mix ½ teaspoon ground ginger with the yogurt in a bowl. Sprinkle with 2–4 tablespoons soft dark brown sugar, according to taste, the oatmeal and 4 tablespoons sultanas. Leave to stand for 5 minutes before serving.

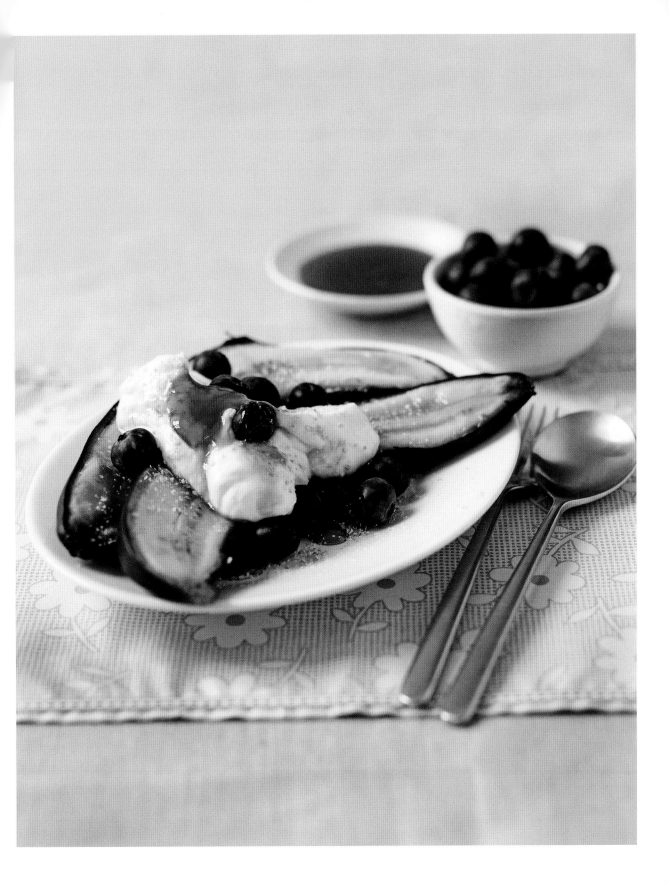

TIP

As well as being rich in vitamin C, this fruit dish provides fibre, phytochemicals and prebiotics as a nourishing treat for your microbiome.

Papaya with Tumbling Berries

2 large papayas

125 g (4 oz) blueberries

125 g (4 oz) raspberries

250 g (8 oz) strawberries, sliced

125 g (4 oz) cherries, pitted (optional)

runny honey, to taste (optional)

lime wedges, to serve

Cut the papayas in half, scoop out the seeds and discard. Place each half on a serving plate.

Mix together the blueberries, raspberries, strawberries and cherries, if using, in a bowl and then pile into the papaya halves. Drizzle with a little honey, if liked, and serve with the lime wedges.

- **FOR PAPAYA & BERRY SMOOTHIE**

Peel and halve the papayas, remove the seeds and cut into chunks. Place in a food processor or blender with the remaining fruits and 10 ice cubes. Add 500 ml (17 fl oz) apple or guava juice and blend until smooth. Pour into glasses and serve immediately.

- **SERVES: 4**
- **PREPARATION TIME: 5 MINUTES, PLUS CHILLING AND STANDING**

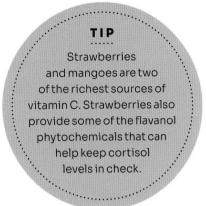

TIP
Strawberries and mangoes are two of the richest sources of vitamin C. Strawberries also provide some of the flavanol phytochemicals that can help keep cortisol levels in check.

Balsamic Strawberries & Mango

500 g (1 lb) strawberries, thickly sliced

1 large mango, peeled, stoned and sliced

1–2 tablespoons caster sugar, to taste

3 tablespoons balsamic vinegar

2 tablespoons chopped mint, to decorate

Mix together the strawberries and mango in a large, shallow bowl, sprinkle with the sugar, according to taste, and pour over the balsamic vinegar. Cover with clingfilm and chill overnight.

Remove the fruit from the refrigerator and leave to stand for at least 1 hour before serving.

Spoon the fruit into serving bowls, drizzle over the juices and serve, sprinkled with the mint.

- **FOR PEPPERY STRAWBERRIES & BLUEBERRIES**

Mix the strawberries with 125 g (4 oz) blueberries and prepare as above. Sprinkle with a few grinds of black pepper and the chopped mint before serving.

- **SERVES: 10**
- **PREPARATION TIME: 15 MINUTES**
- **COOKING TIME: 45–50 MINUTES**

Beetroot Speckled Cake

200 g (7 oz) butter, melted, plus extra for greasing

200 g (7 oz) soft light brown sugar

200 g (7 oz) raw beetroot, peeled and grated

150 g (5 oz) whole mixed nuts, toasted and chopped

3 eggs, separated

1 teaspoon baking powder

½ teaspoon ground cinnamon

grated rind and juice of 1 orange

200 g (7 oz) rice flour

3 tablespoons ground almonds

To decorate

200 g (7 oz) cream cheese

1 tablespoon icing sugar

150 g (5 oz) whole mixed nuts

Grease a 20 cm (8 inch) round deep cake tin.

Whisk together the melted butter and sugar in a large bowl until pale. Stir in the beetroot, two-thirds of the nuts and the egg yolks.

Stir together the baking powder, cinnamon, orange rind and juice, flour and ground almonds in a separate bowl. Add to the beetroot mixture and beat until smooth.

Whisk the egg whites in a large clean bowl until they form soft peaks, then fold into the beetroot mixture.

Spoon the mixture into the prepared tin and place in a preheated oven, 200°C (400°F), Gas Mark 6, for 45–50 minutes until firm to the touch. Remove from the oven and transfer to a wire rack to cool.

Beat together the cream cheese and icing sugar in a bowl, then smooth the icing over the top of the cooled cake. Decorate with the whole nuts.

- **FOR CHOCOLATE BEETROOT CAKE**

Make the cake mixture as above and fold in 100 g (3½ oz) chopped plain dark chocolate. Bake as above and leave to cool. Top the cake with grated chocolate.

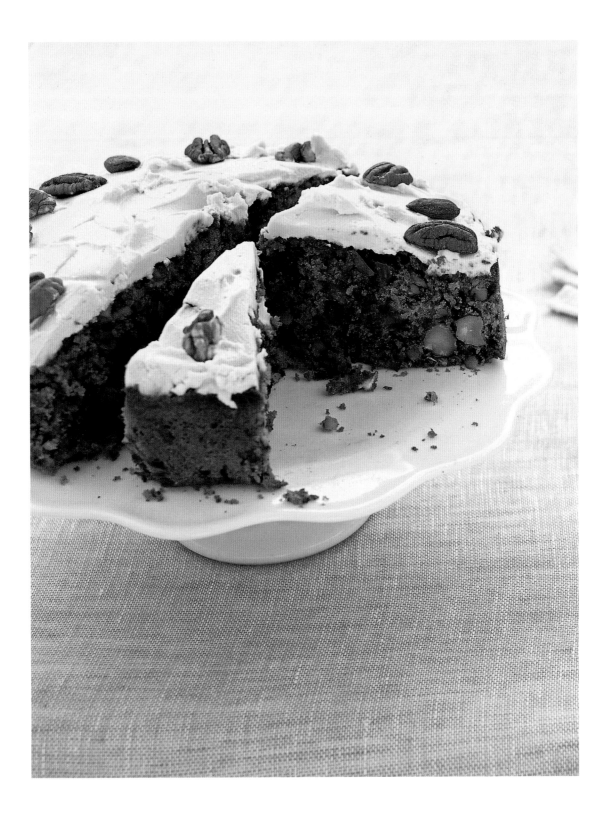

- **SERVES: 4**
- **PREPARATION TIME: 10 MINUTES**
- **COOKING TIME: 45–50 MINUTES**

Pear, Almond & Chocolate Cake

100 ml (3½ fl oz) groundnut oil

125 g (4 oz) fat-free natural yogurt

1 teaspoon vanilla extract

175 g (6 oz) golden caster sugar

225 g (7½ oz) wholemeal flour

50 g (2 oz) ground almonds

2 teaspoons baking powder

pinch of salt

3 eggs, lightly beaten

75 g (3 oz) plain dark chocolate chips

1 large firm, ripe Comice pear, peeled, cored and coarsely grated

100 g (3½ oz) whole blanched almonds (optional)

half-fat crème fraîche, to serve (optional)

Beat together the oil, yogurt, vanilla extract, sugar, flour, ground almonds, baking powder and salt in a large bowl. Add the eggs, one by one, beating well after each addition.

Fold in the chocolate chips and pear and spoon into a deep, round 20 cm (8 inch) nonstick cake tin. Arrange the blanched almonds over the top of the cake, if using.

Place in a preheated oven, 180°C (350°F), Gas Mark 4, for 45–50 minutes or until the cake is risen, golden and firm to the touch.

Leave to cool for 15 minutes in the tin, then remove from the tin and cool completely on a wire rack. Serve in thick wedges with dollops of half-fat crème fraîche, if liked.

- **FOR LIME & BLUEBERRY YOGURT CAKE**

Make as above, replacing the vanilla extract with the grated rind of 1 lime and the pear with 125 g (4 oz) blueberries. Omit the chocolate chips and blanched almonds. Scatter 2 tablespoons grated coconut over the top before baking. Bake as above.

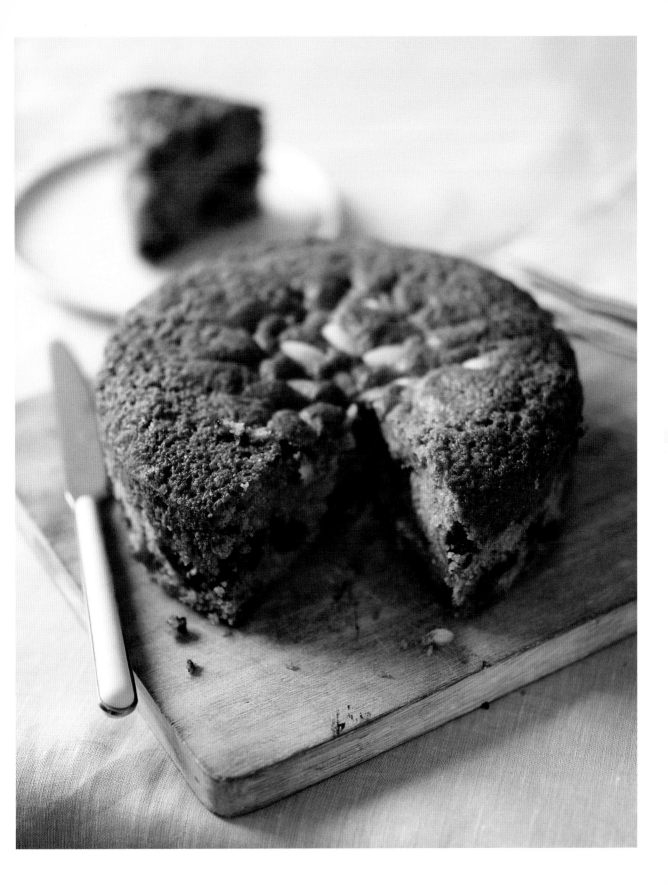

- **SERVES: 4**
- **PREPARATION TIME: 5 MINUTES**
- **COOKING TIME: 25–30 MINUTES**

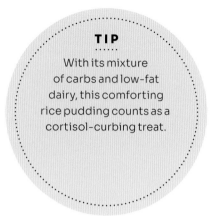

TIP

With its mixture of carbs and low-fat dairy, this comforting rice pudding counts as a cortisol-curbing treat.

Rice Pudding with Toasted Nuts

125 g (4 oz) brown pudding rice

750 ml (1¼ pints) skimmed or semi-skimmed milk

2 cardamom pods, lightly crushed

finely grated rind of ½ lemon

25 g (1 oz) soft dark brown sugar, plus extra to serve (optional)

1 vanilla pod, split in half lengthways

100 g (3½ oz) mixed blanched nuts, such as Brazil nuts, hazelnuts and shelled pistachio nuts

Put the rice in a heavy-based saucepan with the milk, cardamom, lemon rind and sugar. Scrape in the seeds from the vanilla pod and place over a medium heat. Bring to the boil, then reduce the heat, partially cover and simmer very gently, stirring regularly, for 25–30 minutes, or until the rice is tender and creamy, adding more milk if necessary.

Meanwhile, place the nuts in a small freezer bag and tap lightly with a rolling pin until they are crushed but not ground. Tip into a nonstick frying pan and dry-fry over a low heat for 5–6 minutes, stirring continuously, until golden. Tip on to a plate and leave to cool.

Spoon the rice pudding into bowls and sprinkle over a little extra brown sugar, if liked. Scatter over the toasted nuts and serve.

- **FOR RICE PUDDING WITH FRESH FIG COMPOTE**

Cook the rice pudding as above. Put 4 roughly chopped fresh figs and 125 ml (4 fl oz) apple juice in a small pan and simmer gently for 10–12 minutes or until the fruit is tender. Either leave the compote chunky or blend to a purée in a food processor or blender. Serve with the rice pudding.

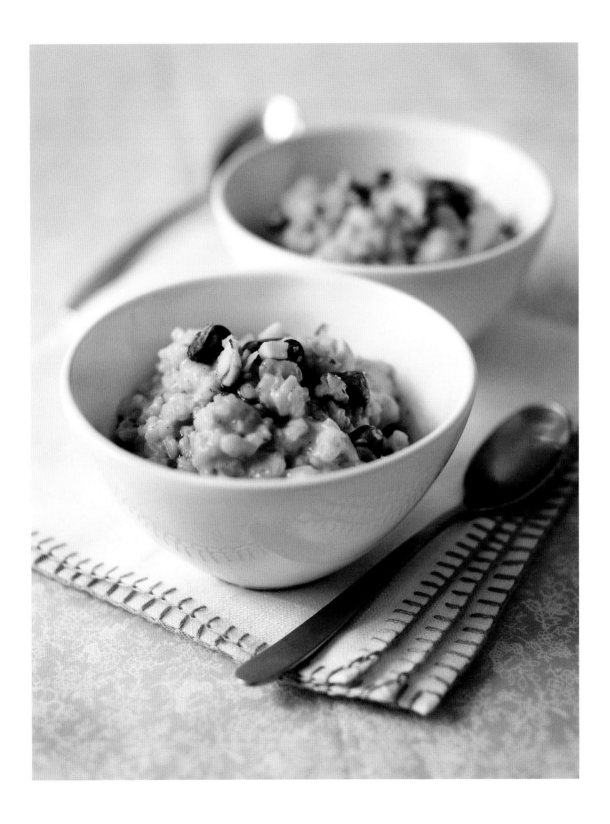

- **SERVES: 4**
- **PREPARATION TIME: 20 MINUTES**
- **COOKING TIME: 20 MINUTES**

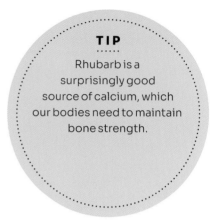

TIP

Rhubarb is a surprisingly good source of calcium, which our bodies need to maintain bone strength.

Rhubarb & Strawberry Salad

500 g (1 lb) rhubarb

125 g (4 oz) caster sugar

150 ml (¼ pint) water

1 vanilla pod

2 teaspoons rosewater

400 g (13 oz) strawberries

To serve

mascarpone cheese or Greek yogurt

40 g (1½ oz) roughly chopped pistachio nuts

Cut the rhubarb into 4 cm (1½ inch) lengths and put them in a shallow, non-metallic ovenproof dish.

Put the sugar and water in a small saucepan over a low heat and stir until the sugar has dissolved. Add the vanilla pod and rosewater. Pour the syrup over the rhubarb, cover with foil and bake in a preheated oven, 180°C (350°F), Gas Mark 4, for 12–15 minutes until just soft.

Meanwhile, hull and halve the strawberries. When the rhubarb is cooked, discard the vanilla pod and add the strawberries, cover and leave to stand for 5 minutes. Transfer the fruit to serving plates, spoon some of the cooking liquid over each one and add a dollop of mascarpone or yogurt and a sprinkling of chopped pistachios.

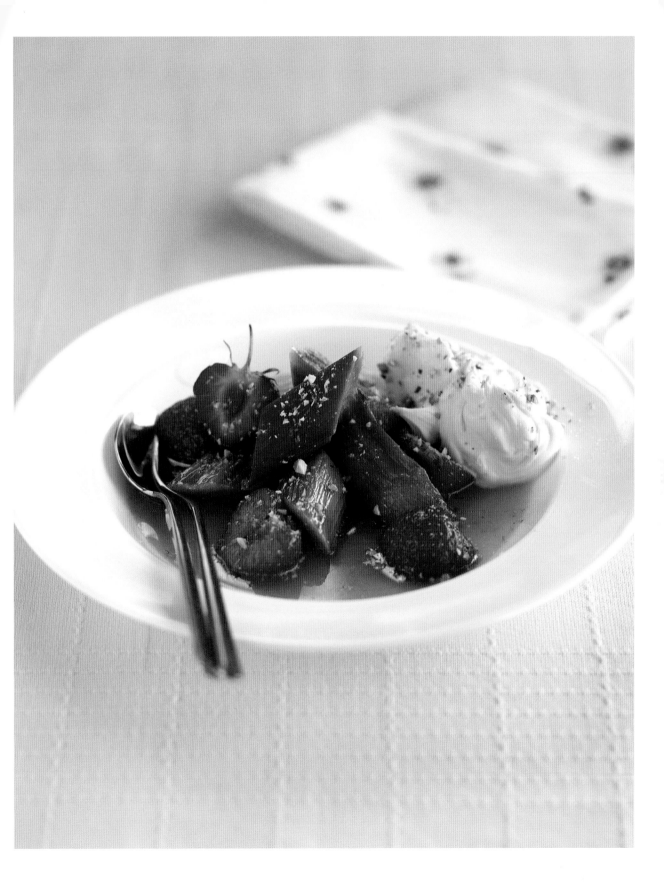

- **SERVES: 4**
- **PREPARATION TIME: 15 MINUTES, PLUS FREEZING**
- **COOKING TIME: 5 MINUTES**

TIP

Choose an orange-fleshed melon such as cantaloupe or Charentais for a higher amount of carotenoids – antioxidants that the body can also turn into vitamin A.

Melon Granita

1 ripe orange-fleshed melon

75 g (3 oz) caster sugar

150 ml (¼ pint) water

2 tablespoons melon liqueur (optional)

Cut the melon in half and remove and discard the seeds, then roughly chop the flesh – you need about 450 g (14½ oz).

Place the caster sugar in a saucepan with the water and stir over a low heat until dissolved, then bring to the boil.

Remove from the heat and leave to cool, then place in a food processor with the chopped melon flesh and melon liqueur, if using. Blend until smooth.

Transfer to a shallow freezer-proof container and freeze for 1 hour or until ice crystals appear at the edges. Stir the ice into the centre and return to the freezer. Stir and refreeze a few more times until the granita is completely frozen.

To serve, scrape the granita with a fork and serve immediately.

Poached Fruit with Ginger Biscuits

....

100g (3½ oz) caster sugar

1.2 litres (2 pints) water

1 vanilla pod

2 peaches

2 nectarines

5 apricots

To serve

mascarpone cheese

1 or 2 ginger biscuits, crushed

Put the sugar, water and vanilla pod in a large, heavy-based saucepan and heat gently, stirring, until the sugar has dissolved. Bring to a low simmer, add the fruit and cover with a circle of baking paper to hold the fruit in the syrup. Simmer for 2 minutes then turn off the heat and leave to cool.

Remove the fruit from the liquid with a slotted spoon, reserving the poaching liquid. Peel the skins from the fruit, then cut them in half and remove the stones.

Put 125 ml (4 fl oz) of the poaching liquid in a small, heavy-based saucepan and simmer for 6–8 minutes until it has a syrupy consistency. Put the fruit in a large bowl, pour over the syrup and toss gently. Arrange the fruit on serving plates, add a spoonful of mascarpone to each one and sprinkle with crushed ginger biscuits.

- **SERVES: 4–6**
- **PREPARATION TIME: 10 MINUTES**
- **COOKING TIME: 20 MINUTES**

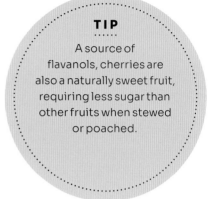

TIP

A source of flavanols, cherries are also a naturally sweet fruit, requiring less sugar than other fruits when stewed or poached.

Cherries with Cinnamon Crumble

1.5 kg (3 lb) frozen pitted dark cherries

1 tablespoon sugar

4 tablespoons water

1 vanilla pod

2 cloves

pared zest of 1 orange

Crumble

60 g (2¼ oz) ready-made fruit loaf

15 g (½ oz) unsalted butter

⅛ teaspoon ground cinnamon

1 tablespoon caster sugar

crème fraîche, to serve

Put the cherries (still frozen is fine) in a large saucepan with the sugar, water, vanilla pod, cloves and orange zest. Bring to a slow simmer, stirring occasionally, then when thoroughly piping hot all the way through turn off the heat and leave covered.

Meanwhile, make the crumble. Cut the fruit loaf into 1 cm (½ inch) dice. Melt the butter and drizzle it over the fruit loaf. Mix together the cinnamon and sugar and sprinkle over the fruit loaf. Mix well, transfer to a baking sheet and cook in a preheated oven, 190°C (375°F), Gas Mark 5, for 4–5 minutes until golden and crunchy. Remove the crumble from the oven and allow to cool a little.

Serve the warm cherries topped with the crumble and a little crème fraîche.

- **FOR CHERRIES WITH CHOCOLATE & CINNAMON SAUCE**

Combine 100 g (3½ oz) chopped dark chocolate (with 70 per cent cocoa solids), 15 g (½ oz) butter, 125 ml (4 fl oz) cream and ½ teaspoon ground cinnamon in a small, heavy-based saucepan over a low heat. Stir the sauce until all the chocolate has melted and it is smooth and glossy. Turn off the heat and reserve. Prepare the cherries as above and serve with a drizzle of the chocolate cinnamon sauce.

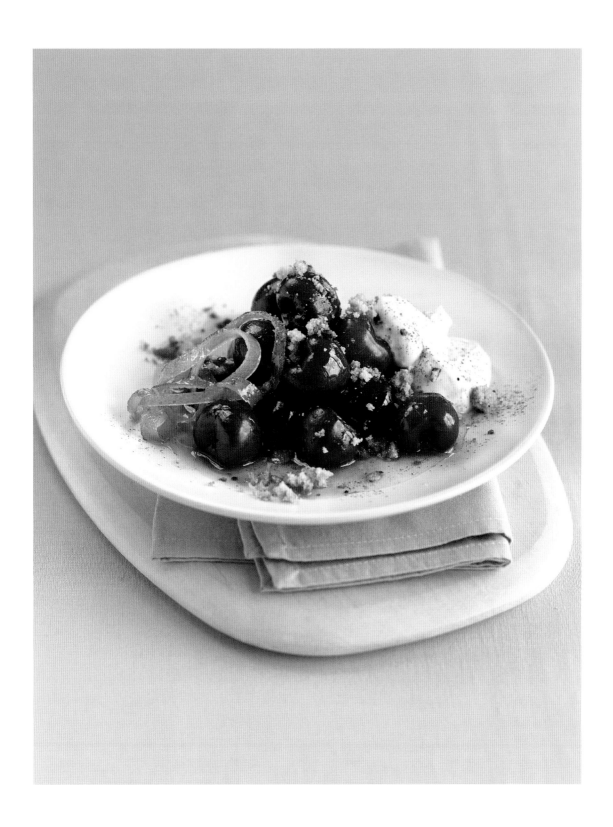

- SERVES: 6–8
- PREPARATION TIME: 6 MINUTES
- COOKING TIME: 3 MINUTES

TIP

This is definitely a treat dessert (perhaps for a dinner party), but don't feel too guilty because dark chocolate and cocoa provide cortisol-friendly flavanols.

Chocolate Mint Mascarpone Tart

200 g (7 oz) dark chocolate with mint crisp, broken into small pieces

150 g (5 oz) mascarpone cheese

100 ml (3½ fl oz) double cream

20 cm (8 inch) ready-made sweet pastry case

mint leaves, to decorate

To serve

crème fraîche

cocoa powder

Melt the chocolate in a heatproof bowl set over a pan of gently simmering water, then leave to cool slightly.

Whip the mascarpone and cream with a hand-held electric whisk until smooth and thickened. Stir in the melted chocolate until well combined, then spoon into the pastry case.

Decorate with mint leaves and serve in slices with spoonfuls of crème fraîche and a dusting of cocoa.

- **FOR CHOCOLATE & CHILLI FONDUE**

Place 200 g (7 oz) chilli-flavoured dark chocolate, broken into small pieces, in a heatproof bowl with 300 ml (½ pint) double cream and 25 g (1 oz) unsalted butter. Set over a pan of gently simmering water and heat gently for 5–7 minutes, stirring occasionally, until the mixture is smooth and glossy. Transfer to a fondue pot or warmed bowl and serve immediately with marshmallows and a selection of fruit, such as bananas and strawberries, for dipping.

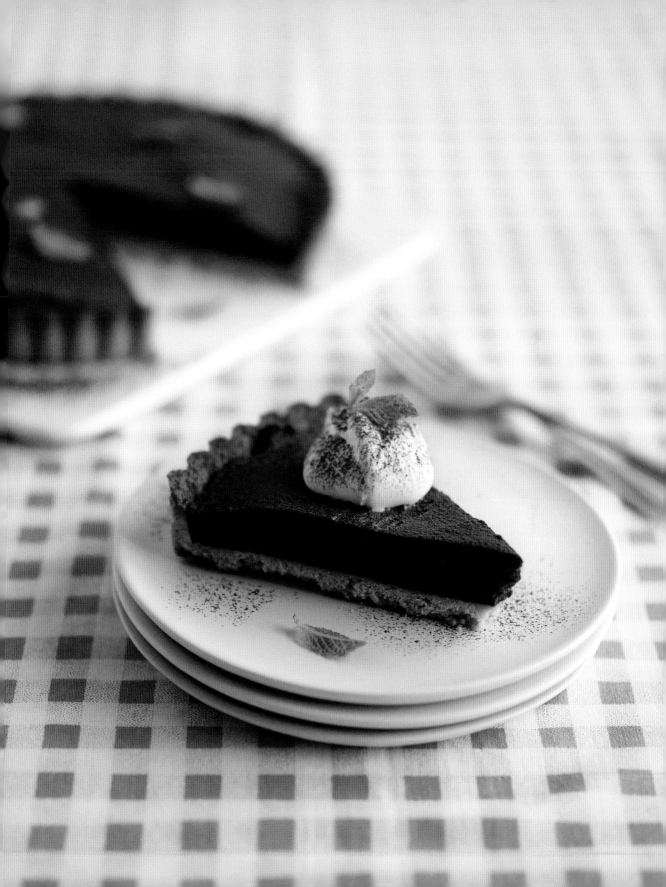

- **SERVES: 4**
- **PREPARATION TIME: 15 MINUTES**
- **COOKING TIME: 15 MINUTES**

Banana & Fig Filo Pastry

6 large sheets of filo pastry

50 g (2 oz) unsalted butter, melted

4 bananas, sliced

6 dried figs, sliced

25 g (1 oz) caster sugar (optional)

grated rind of ½ lemon

½ teaspoon ground cinnamon

thick double cream or Greek yogurt, to serve

Cut the pastry sheets in half crossways. Lay one sheet flat on a baking sheet and brush with melted butter, top with a second sheet and again brush with melted butter. Repeat with the remaining sheets.

Arrange the banana and fig slices over the pastry. Combine the sugar (if using), lemon rind and cinnamon, then sprinkle over the fruit and drizzle over any remaining melted butter.

Bake in a preheated oven, 200°C (400°F), Gas Mark 6, for 15 minutes until the pastry is crisp and the fruit golden. Serve hot with cream or Greek yogurt.

- **FOR SPICED APPLE FILO PASTRY**

Prepare the filo pastry base as above. Core and quarter 2 apples and cut into wafer-thin slices. Arrange the slices over the pastry in overlapping rows. Drizzle over 25 g (1 oz) melted butter and sprinkle with 2 tablespoons caster sugar mixed with 1 teaspoon ground cinnamon. Bake as above for 20 minutes.

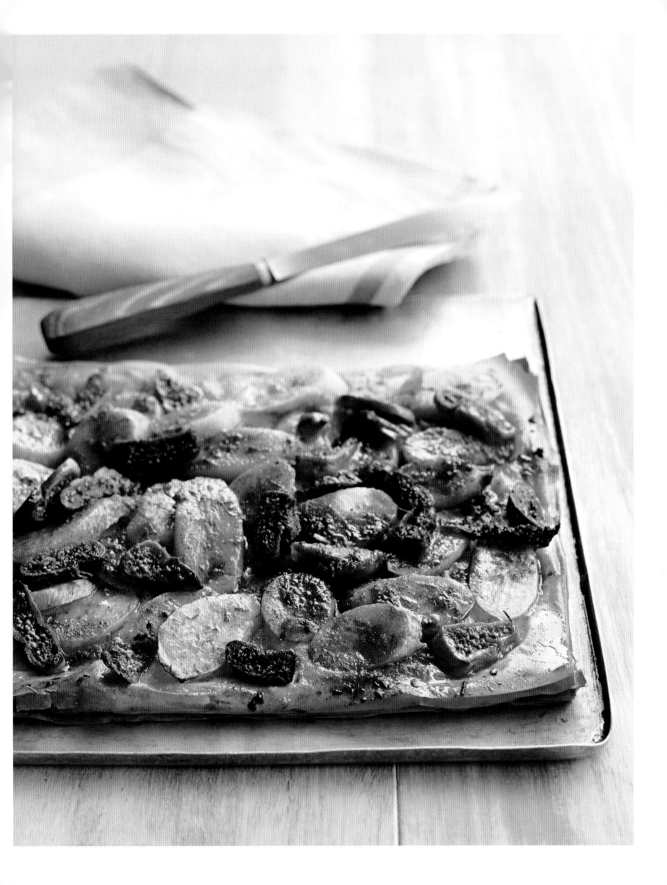

Lemon Cookies

....

125 ml (4 fl oz) olive oil

4 tablespoons soya yogurt

juice of 1 lemon

grated rind of 3 lemons

125 g (4 oz) light muscovado sugar

165 g (5½ oz) plain flour

75 g (3 oz) rolled oats

40 g (1½ oz) millet flakes

40 g (1½ oz) desiccated coconut,
plus 1 tablespoon for dusting

Mix together the olive oil, yogurt, lemon juice and grated rind of 2 lemons in a bowl. In a separate bowl, mix together the sugar, flour, oats, millet flakes and coconut.

Stir the wet ingredients into the dry ingredients and mix to form a soft dough.

Roll the dough into 20 balls, then place on a baking sheet and press down gently. Sprinkle the cookies with the extra desiccated coconut and the remaining lemon rind.

Bake in a preheated oven, 180°C (350°F), Gas Mark 4, for 12–15 minutes until golden. Leave to cool on the sheet for a few minutes, then transfer to a wire rack and leave to cool completely. Store in an airtight container and eat within 2–3 days.

....

- **FOR LEMON POSSET**

Mix together 400 g (13 oz) fat-free Greek yogurt, 1 tablespoon icing sugar, the grated rind of 3 lemons and 2 teaspoons lemon juice in a bowl. Spoon into 4 small glasses or bowls and chill for at least 1 hour. Sprinkle 1 tablespoon desiccated coconut over the possets, then serve each with 1 lemon cookie (see above).

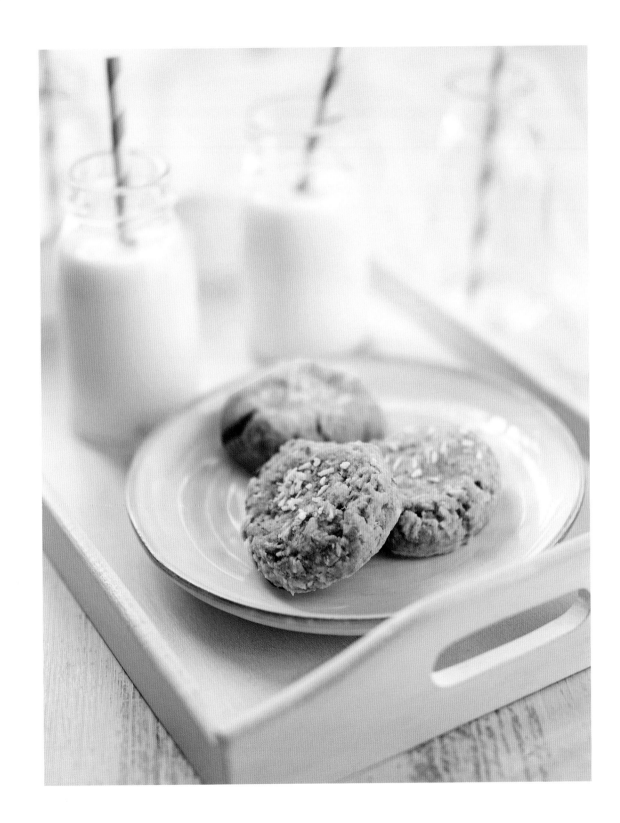

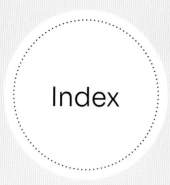

Index

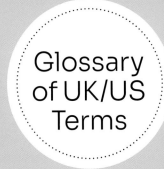

Glossary of UK/US Terms

UK	US
aubergine	eggplant
baking paper	waxed or parchment paper
baking sheet	cookie sheet
beetroot	beet
bicarbonate of soda	baking soda
biscuit	cookie
broad bean	fava or lima bean
cake tin	baking tin, cake pan
caster sugar	superfine sugar
chickpea	garbanzo bean
chilli	chili or chile pepper
clingfilm	plastic wrap
coriander (chopped, sprigs, leaves)	cilantro
cornmeal	polenta
courgette	zucchini
crumble (fruit crumble)	fruit crisp
dark chocolate	semi-sweet chocolate
desiccated coconut	shredded coconut
dessert apple	sweet apple
double cream	heavy cream
flaked almonds	slivered almonds
foil	aluminum foil
frying pan	skillet
grated	shredded
green beans	string beans
grill, to grill	broiler, to broil
groundnut oil	peanut oil
icing	frosting
icing sugar	confectioner's or powdered sugar
jug	pitcher
kitchen paper	paper towel
lemon rind	lemon peel
mangetout	snow pea
natural yogurt	unflavoured yogurt
orange rind	orange peel
pastry case	pie shell
pepper (red, orange, yellow, green)	bell pepper
plain flour	all-purpose flour
porridge oats	oatmeal
prawn	shrimp
rapeseed oil	canola oil
self-raising flour	self-rising flour
semi-skimmed milk	2% milk
skimmed milk	non-fat milk
spring onion	scallion
starter	appetizer
stoned	pitted, seeded
sultana	yellow raisin
tomato purée	tomato paste
unsalted butter	sweet butter
wholemeal	wholewheat

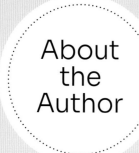

About the Author

Angela Dowden is a UK Registered Nutritionist and freelance health writer and author. She has over 20 years' expertise writing for national newspapers and magazines, including several years as a columnist at both *WOMAN* and *Woman's Own*. Her nutrition philosophy is that one size doesn't fit all, and that a healthy diet should be fad-free and tasty.

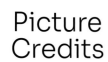

Picture Credits

Octopus Publishing Group: Frank Adam 55; Stephen Conroy 43, 151, 195; Will Heap 107, 171; William Lingwood 23, 177; David Munns 137, 141, 145, 173; Emma Neish 47, 201; William Reavell 129; Lis Parsons 51, 57, 69, 71, 73, 75, 77, 79, 85, 133, 139, 169, 207, 211; William Shaw 19, 21, 29, 33, 37, 39, 41, 59, 65, 67, 89, 91, 93, 95, 100, 103, 105, 111, 113, 117, 119, 123, 125, 127, 135, 143, 147, 149, 153, 157, 159, 161, 175, 181, 183, 185, 187, 189, 193, 197, 203, 205, 213, 217; Ian Wallace 27, 31, 45, 61, 165, 167, 215; Philip Webb 81.